OVERVIEW-MAP KEY

● ●

rk

ark

:: OTHER BOOKS BY JOHNNY MOLLOY

50 Hikes in Alabama

50 Hikes in the Ozarks

50 Hikes in the North Georgia Mountains

50 Hikes in South Carolina

50 Hikes on Tennessee's Cumberland Plateau

60 Hikes Within 60 Miles: San Antonio & Austin (with Tom Taylor)

60 Hikes Within 60 Miles: Nashville

A Canoeing & Kayaking Guide to the Streams of Florida

A Canoeing & Kayaking Guide to the Streams of Kentucky (with Bob Sehlinger)

A Paddler's Guide to Everglades National Park

Backcountry Fishing: A Guide for Hikers, Backpackers and Paddlers

Beach & Coastal Camping in Florida

Beach & Coastal Camping in the Southeast

Best Easy Day Hikes: Cincinnati

Best East Day Hikes: Greensboro/ Winston-Salem

Best Easy Day Hikes: Jacksonville

Best Easy Day Hikes: Madison, Wisconsin

Best Easy Day Hikes: New River Gorge

Best Easy Day Hikes: Richmond

Best Easy Day Hikes: Tallahassee

Best Easy Day Hikes: Tampa Bay

Best Hikes Near Cincinnati

Best Hikes Near Columbus

Best Tent Camping: The Carolinas

Best Tent Camping: Colorado

Best Tent Camping: Kentucky

Best Tent Camping: Southern Appalachian & Smoky Mountains

Best Tent Camping: Tennessee

Best Tent Camping: West Virginia

Best Tent Camping: Wisconsin

Can't Miss Hikes in North Carolina's National Forests

Day & Overnight Hikes on Kentucky's Sheltowee Trace

Day & Overnight Hikes in West Virginia's Monongahela National Forest

Day Hiking Southwest Florida

Five-Star Trails: Chattanooga

Five-Star Trails: Knoxville

Five-Star Trails: Tri-Cities Tennessee and Virginia

From the Swamp to the Keys: A Paddle through Florida History

Hiking the Florida Trail: 1,100 Miles, 78 Days and Two Pairs of Boots

Hiking Mississippi

Hiking Through History: New England

Hiking Through History: Virginia

Mount Rogers National Recreation Area Guidebook

The Hiking Trails of Florida's National Forests, Parks, and Preserves

Land Between the Lakes Outdoor Recreation Handbook

Long Trails of the Southeast

Outward Bound Canoeing Handbook

Paddling Georgia

Paddling South Carolina

Paddling Tennessee

Top Trails: Great Smoky Mountains National Park

Top Trails: Shenandoah National Park

Trial By Trail: Backpacking in the Smoky Mountains

Waterfall Hiking Tennessee

Waterfalls of the Blue Ridge

Visit the author's website at **johnnymolloy.com**

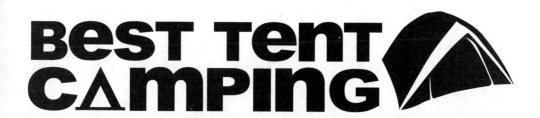

BEST TENT CAMPING

GEORGIA

YOUR CAR-CAMPING GUIDE TO SCENIC BEAUTY, THE SOUNDS OF NATURE, AND AN ESCAPE FROM CIVILIZATION

Third Edition

JOHNNY MOLLOY

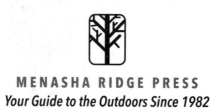

MENASHA RIDGE PRESS
Your Guide to the Outdoors Since 1982

: *This book is for my pal Ken Ashley, who has spent many a night camping in Georgia.*

Best Tent Camping: Georgia, 3rd Edition

Copyright © 2014 by Johnny Molloy
All rights reserved
Printed in the United States of America
Published by Menasha Ridge Press
Distributed by the Publishers Group West
Third edition, first printing

Molloy, Johnny, 1961-
  Best tent camping. Georgia : your car-camping guide to scenic beauty, the sounds of nature, and an escape from civilization / Johnny Molloy. — Third edition.
     pages cm — (Best tent camping)
  ISBN 978-0-89732-498-4 (paperback) — ISBN 978-0-89732-499-1 (eISBN)
  1. Camping—Georgia—Guidebooks. 2. Camp sites, facilities, etc.—Georgia—Guidebooks. 3. Georgia—Guidebooks. I. Title.
  GV191.42.G4 M65
  796.5409758—dc23

                    2014033610

Cover design by Scott McGrew
Cover photo © Pat & Chuck Blackley / Alamy
Text design by Annie Long
Cartography by Steve Jones and Johnny Molloy
Indexing by Rich Carlson

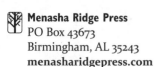 **Menasha Ridge Press**
PO Box 43673
Birmingham, AL 35243
menasharidgepress.com

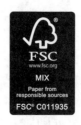

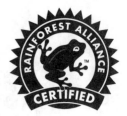

CONTENTS

• •

:: MIDDLE GEORGIA   109

:: SOUTH GEORGIA   134

:: APPENDIXES AND INDEX   165

BEST CAMPGROUNDS

ACKNOWLEDGMENTS

● ●

I would like to thank the following people for helping me in the research and writing of this book: all the land managers of Georgia's state parks and forests and the folks at Oconee and Chattahoochee National Forests and Cumberland Island National Seashore. Also, many thanks to the administrators at the Army Corps of Engineers. More thanks go to the campground hosts who are on the ground at all the campgrounds throughout the state.

Thanks to my wife, Keri Anne, for her help. Thanks to Levi Novey for camping with me on the Jacks River and for lending his thoughts on the future of the outdoors and of our national parks and forests. Thanks to Cisco Meyer for checking the radar and camping all over the mountains through the years, from Mountaintown Creek to Amicalola Falls to the Cohutta Wilderness. Thanks to Sierra Designs for providing me with excellent tents, sleeping bags, and outerwear. Thanks to John Cox for camping with me in northern Georgia and Wes Shepherd down south. The biggest thanks of all goes to the people of Georgia, who have a beautiful state in which to tent camp.

PREFACE

● ●

Welcome to the 3rd edition of this book. Exploring the mountains of northern Georgia was a natural extension of my camping, hiking, and paddling obsession that began in the Smoky Mountains more than three decades ago. My very first trip in Georgia was to Cloudland Canyon, led by Calvin Milam. We camped and explored the trails and vistas that opened my eyes to all the possibilities here. More trips covered the Cohutta Mountains and the ridges where the Appalachian Trail headed from Springer Mountain toward its ultimate destination in Maine.

Later, I moved to Atlanta, and adventuring in Georgia became much easier. I explored the mountains from top to bottom and also began canoeing down many of the state's rivers, from the Etowah to the Flint to the Satilla, and waterways beyond. More trips led south, to Cumberland Island National Seashore and the one and only Okefenokee Swamp. I have made repeated trips to these south Georgia treasures, paddling along the dark water trails of the swamp that contrast mightily with the open, sandy Atlantic shoreline of Cumberland Island.

Time passed, and I began writing outdoor guidebooks—"camping for keeps," if you will. The opportunity arose to write this guidebook, and I jumped on it excitedly and began systematically exploring the Georgia landscape for the best tent campgrounds in the state. The first surprise came at Cotton Hill, an Army Corps of Engineers campground on Lake Eufaula. The walk-in tent campsites offered first-rate waterfront camping with knockout views. Next, I headed to Kolomoki Mounds in southwest Georgia and delved into the past of this land, inspecting the largest Indian mounds east of the Mississippi River. Kolomoki Mounds demonstrate that human and natural history, as well as quality outdoor recreation, are important components of the best tent campgrounds in Georgia. River Junction Campground on Lake Seminole provided further evidence that the Peach State's abundant lakes offer watery recreation from top to bottom. It was hard to pick the best among all of Georgia's large lakes, much less the smaller ones, like Lake Winfield Scott, a serene mountain impoundment in the Chattahoochee National Forest, where no gas motors are allowed. In many places, well-located campgrounds allowed both water and land recreation, like Rood Creek Campground, near Providence Canyon State Park, known as Georgia's "Little Grand Canyon." Since the first two editions of this book, I have also written hiking and paddling guides for the state, expanding my knowledge of Georgia outdoors, which has enabled me to share that information with you.

The Peach State has some of the most appealing coastline in America, with its large rivers following gravity, mixing in with salt water, melding into the marsh islands and sea islands of the Atlantic Ocean. I especially enjoyed Fort McAllister State Park, with its campground on a small sea island and fascinating Civil War fort, which Confederate General Robert E. Lee helped design. Speaking of history, anyone who hasn't visited the F. D. Roosevelt State Park is missing out on a brilliant melding of beauty and history atop Pine Mountain in middle Georgia near Columbus. Here, the campground serves as a base camp for walks on the Pine Mountain Trail, to see rustic stone buildings that are works of the Civilian Conservation Corps. Magnolia Springs State Park is another regional treasure. The spring itself, brilliant blue to behold, also has a place in Civil War history.

After many camping trips and many, many nights under the stars, this list of the 50 best campgrounds began to fill, and, finally, I determined the last "winner" (so many campgrounds did not make the state's top 50). And with the joy of completing a book and the sadness of an adventure ended, I finished my research. In writing and updating new editions of this guide, I have continued to put my knowledge to work, enjoying more of the Georgia outdoors. I'll look out for you at the campground, on the river, or out on the trail!

INTRODUCTION

● ●

A Word about This Book and Georgia Tent Camping

I am grateful for the opportunity to update and revise this book, for it gave me yet another chance to explore the Peach State. In this edition, you will find excellent campgrounds to visit and updated information on every campground contained within. This way, it'll keep the surprises to a minimum. (I still can't control the weather for your tent-camping adventures.) Georgia is rich in both human and natural history. Originally settled by Native Americans from the mountains in the north to the swamps in the south, the area was colonized by a budding United States, starting on the coast and heading inland. The beauty of the coastline was evident in places such as Cumberland Island, but there was more allure inland, where black-water rivers drained the sand-ridge forests of the midlands. Settlers followed the Chattahoochee River from its lower reaches to the headwaters deep in the mountains.

The vast and varied landscape was evident to all who came to Georgia. Today, tent campers can enjoy these parcels, each a distinct region of the state. You can camp on a genuine sea island at Fort McAllister State Park. The sand-ridge forests are well represented at General Coffee State Park, where the Seventeen Mile River slips silently beneath a swamp forest. The ridge and valley country of northwest Georgia stands out at Cloudland Canyon State Park, where vertical stone bluffs allow vistas into deep chasms. The mountains of northeast Georgia, home of the Chattahoochee National Forest, offer recreation destinations aplenty, from streamside trout fishing venues on the Toccoa River to camps adjacent to wilderness areas, such as Tate Branch, to high-country destinations where the summers are cool, such as Black Rock Mountain State Park. Georgia is blessed with lakes aplenty from Lake Seminole on the Florida border, where Spanish moss sways from the lakeside forests, to Lake Hartwell, a busy and large recreation lake in the Savannah River basin. And there's Lake Conasauga in the northwest, an impoundment 3,400 feet in elevation. More lakes await throughout the state.

All this spells paradise for the tent camper. No matter where you go, the scenery will never fail to please the eye. And outdoor activities are plentiful, from canoeing, fishing, hiking, swimming, and boating to just relaxing around the campfire. Before embarking on a trip, take time to prepare. Many of the best tent campgrounds are a fair distance from the civilized world, and you want to be enjoying yourself rather than making supply or gear runs. Call ahead and ask for a park map, brochure, or other information to help you plan your trip. Visit the Web sites listed in this guidebook. Make reservations wherever applicable, especially at popular state parks. Inquire about the latest reservation fees and entrance fees at state parks and forests.

Ask questions. Ask more questions. Although this guide is an indispensable tool for the Georgia-bound camper, the more questions you ask, the fewer surprises you will get. There are other times, however, when you'll grab your gear and this book, hop in the car, and just wing it. This can be an adventure in its own right.

How to Use This Guidebook

We at Menasha Ridge Press welcome you to *Best Tent Camping Georgia*. Whether you're new to this activity or you've been sleeping in your portable outdoor shelter over decades of outdoor adventures, please review the following information. It explains how we have worked with the author to organize this book and how you can make the best use of it.

:: THE RATINGS & RATING CATEGORIES

As with all of the books in the publisher's *Best Tent Camping* series, this guidebook's author personally experienced dozens of campgrounds and campsites to select the top 50 locations in this region. Within that universe of 50 sites, the author then ranked each one in the six categories described below. Each campground in this guidebook is superlative in its own way. For example, a site may be rated only one star in one category but perhaps five stars in another category. This rating system allows you to choose your destination based on the attributes that are most important to you. Though these ratings are subjective, they're still excellent guidelines for finding the perfect camping experience for you and your companions. Below and following, we describe the criteria for each of the attributes in our five-star rating system:

★ ★ ★ ★ ★   The site is **ideal** in that category.

★ ★ ★ ★   The site is **exemplary** in that category.

★ ★ ★   The site is **very good** in that category.

★ ★   The site is **above average** in that category.

★   The site is **acceptable** in that category.

Beauty

In the best campgrounds, the fluid shapes and elements of nature—flora, water, land, and sky—have melded to create locales that seem to have been made especially for tent camping. The best sites are so attractive you may be tempted to not leave your outdoor home. A little site work is all right to make the scenic area camper-friendly, but too many reminders of civilization eliminated many a campground from inclusion in this book.

Privacy

A little understory goes a long way in making you feel comfortable once you've picked your site for the night. There is a trend in planting natural borders between campsites if the borders don't already exist. With some trees or brush to define each site, everyone has some personal space. That way you can go about the pleasures of tent camping without keeping up with the Joneses at the site next door—or them with you.

Spaciousness

This attribute can be very important depending on the size of your group and how much gear you carry. Campers with family-style tents and screen shelters need a large, flat spot on which to pitch their tent and still get to the ice chest to prepare meals, all while not getting burned near the fire ring. Gearheads need adequate space to show off their portable glow-in-the-dark lounge chairs and other pricey gee-gaws to neighbors strolling by. I just need enough room to keep my bedroom, den, and kitchen separate.

Quiet

Singing birds, rushing streams, waves lapping against a shoreline, wind whooshing through treetops—those are noises tent campers associate with natural Georgia. From bubbling mountain streams to the Atlantic surf, Georgia's best campgrounds offer a quaint and relaxing soundtrack to camouflage the sounds you don't want to hear—autos coming and going, loud neighbors, and so on.

Security

Campground security is relative. A remote campground with no civilization nearby is usually safe, but don't tempt potential thieves by leaving your valuables out for all to see. Use common sense, and go with your instincts. Campground hosts are wonderful to have around, and state parks with locked gates are ideal for security. Get to know your neighbors and develop a buddy system to watch each other's belongings when possible.

Cleanliness

I'm a stickler for this one. Nothing will sabotage a scenic campground like trash. Most of the campgrounds in this guidebook are clean. More rustic campgrounds—my favorite kind—usually receive less maintenance. Busy weekends and holidays will show their effects; however, don't let a little litter spoil your good time. Help clean up, and think of it as doing your part for Georgia's natural environment.

:: THE CAMPGROUND PROFILE

Each profile contains a concise but informative narrative of the campground, as well as individual sites. Not only is the property described, but also readers can get a general idea of the recreational opportunities available—what's in the area and perhaps suggestions for touristy activities. This descriptive text is enhanced with three helpful sidebars: Ratings, Key Information, and Getting There (accurate driving directions that lead you to the campground from the nearest major roadway, along with GPS coordinates).

:: THE OVERVIEW MAP, MAP KEY, AND LEGEND

Use the overview map on the inside front cover to assess the exact locations of each campground. Each campground's number appears on the overview map, on the map key facing the overview map, and in the Table of Contents. It's easy to locate a campground's full profile by flipping through the book and watching for the campground number at the top of each page.

The book is organized by region as indicated in the Table of Contents. A map legend that details the symbols found on the campground layout maps appears on the inside back cover.

:: CAMPGROUND-LAYOUT MAPS

Each profile contains a detailed campground layout map that provides an overhead look at campground sites, internal roads, facilities, and other key items.

:: GPS CAMPGROUND-ENTRANCE COORDINATES

This book includes the GPS coordinates for each campground. Latitude/longitude coordinates tell you where you are by locating a point west (latitude) of the 0° meridian line that passes through Greenwich, England, and north or south of the 0° (longitude) line that belts the Earth, aka the equator.

Topographic maps show latitude/longitude. The survey datum used to arrive at the coordinates in this book is WGS84 (versus NAD27 or WGS83). For readers who own a GPS unit, whether a handheld or onboard device, the latitude/longitude coordinates provided on the first page of each profile may be entered into the GPS unit. Just make sure your GPS device is set to navigate using WGS84 data. Now you can navigate directly to the campground. For more on GPS technology, visit **usgs.gov.**

That said, however, readers can easily find all campgrounds in this book by using the directions given and the campground-layout map, which shows at least one major road leading into the area. But for those who enjoy using the latest GPS technology or their smart phone to navigate, the necessary data has been provided.

:: WEATHER

Georgia's generally temperate climate varies from the wooded mountains to the beaches. Seasonal variation increases as you head upstate and is influenced by Georgia's proximity to the Atlantic Ocean and the Gulf of Mexico. Spring, the most variable season, creeps upon the Peach State starting in late February; winter- and summerlike temperatures are not uncommon this time of year. As summer approaches, the strong fronts weaken and thunderstorms become more frequent as the "three Hs"—heat, haze, and humidity—prevail. In fall, continental fronts once again sweep through, clearing the air and bringing warm days and cool nights, but rain is always possible. Winter works its way south from the mountains, though the entire state often experiences Artic blasts. Georgia averages 40 to 50 inches of rain each year; in addition, the Atlantic and the Gulf frequently bring in tropical storms that can dump inches at a time from June through November.

:: FIRST-AID KIT

A typical first-aid kit may contain more items than you might think necessary. These are just the basics. Prepackaged kits in waterproof bags (Atwater Carey and Adventure Medical make a variety of kits) are available. As a preventive measure, take along sunscreen and insect repellent. Even though there are quite a few items listed here, they pack down into a small space:

- Ace bandages or Spenco joint wraps

- Adhesive bandages, such as Band-Aids

- Antibiotic ointment (Neosporin or the generic equivalent)

- Antiseptic or disinfectant, such as Betadine or hydrogen peroxide

- Aspirin, acetaminophen, or ibuprofen

- Benadryl or the generic equivalent, diphenhydramine (in case of allergic reactions)

- Butterfly-closure bandages

- Comb and tweezers (for removing ticks from your skin)

- Epinephrine in a prefilled syringe (for severe allergic reactions to such things as bee stings)

- Gauze (one roll and six 4-by-4-inch compress pads)

- LED flashlight or headlamp

- Matches or lighter

- Moist towelettes

- Moleskin/Spenco 2nd Skin

- Pocketknife or multipurpose tool

- Waterproof first-aid tape

- Whistle (it's more effective in signaling rescuers than your voice)

:: ANIMAL AND PLANT HAZARDS

Ticks

Ticks like to hang out in the brush that grows around campsites and along trails. Their numbers seem to explode in the hot summer months, but you should be tick-aware during all months of the year. Ticks, which are arthropods and not insects, need a host to feast on in order to reproduce. The ticks that light onto you will be very small, sometimes so tiny that you won't be able to spot them. Primarily of two varieties, deer ticks and dog ticks, both need a few hours of actual attachment before they can transmit any disease they may harbor. Ticks may settle in shoes, socks, and hats, and may take several hours to actually latch on. The best strategy is to visually check yourself a couple of times a day, especially if you've gone out for a walk in the woods. Ticks that haven't attached are easily removed, but not easily killed. If you pick off a tick in the woods, just toss it aside. If you find one on your body at camp, you may want to dispatch it (otherwise it may find you again). For ticks that have embedded, removal with tweezers is best.

Snakes

Georgia has more than 42 snake species—more than any other state. Most are nonpoisonous, but in the mountains watch for the timber rattlesnake and copperhead. Copperheads lurk near streams and on outcrops, whereas rattlers can primarily be found sunning themselves on rocks. Farther south you may see eastern diamondbacks in palmetto stands and pine woods. These snakes are distinguished by their brown-and-yellow diamond pattern; the tail is solid black with rattles. Pygmy rattlers, dull gray and a little more than a foot long, are uncommon but may be found in wet areas and oak—pine woods. Cottonmouths, also known as water moccasins, are found in every type of wetland habitat down south, including estuaries, tidal creeks, and salt marshes. Adults, usually drab brown or olive with darker cross bands, reach lengths of three to four feet and are often heavy bodied. The harmless brown water snake, which is very common in aquatic areas frequented by humans, is often mistaken for the cottonmouth. A key way to tell the difference: water snakes flee when disturbed (cottonmouths stand their ground and assume an open-mouthed warning posture). The Eastern coral snake is a rare sight indeed but is easily identified by the alternating red, yellow, and black rings that encircle its body.

Poison Ivy, Poison Oak, & Poison Sumac

Recognizing poison ivy, oak, and sumac and avoiding contact with them is the most effective way to prevent the painful, itchy rashes associated with these plants. In the Southeast, poison ivy ranges from a thick, tree-hugging vine to a shaded ground cover, three leaflets to a leaf; poison oak occurs as either a vine or shrub, with three leaflets as well; and poison sumac flourishes in swampland, each leaf containing 7 to 13 leaflets. Urushiol, the oil in the sap of these plants, is responsible for the rash. Usually within 12 to 14 hours of exposure (but sometimes much later), raised lines and/or blisters will appear, accompanied by a terrible itch. Refrain from scratching because bacteria under fingernails can cause infection and you will spread the rash to other parts of your body. Wash and dry the rash thoroughly, applying a calamine lotion or other product to help dry the rash. If itching or blistering is severe, seek medical attention. Remember that oil-contaminated clothes, pets, or hiking gear can easily cause an irritating rash on you or someone else, so wash not only any exposed parts of your body but also clothes, gear, and pets.

Mosquitoes

Although it's not a common occurrence, individuals can become infected with the West Nile virus by being bitten by an infected mosquito. Culex mosquitoes, the primary variety that can transmit West Nile virus to humans, thrive in urban rather than natural areas. They lay their eggs in stagnant water and can breed in any standing water that remains for more than five days. Most people infected with West Nile virus have no symptoms of illness, but some may become ill, usually 3 to 15 days after being bitten.

In the mountains, summertime is when mosquitoes are their most troublesome. At this time of year—and anytime you expect mosquitoes to be buzzing around—you may want to wear protective clothing, such as long sleeves, long pants, and socks. Loose-fitting, light-colored clothing is best. Spray clothing with insect repellent. Remember to follow the instructions on the repellent and to take extra care with children.

:: TIPS FOR A HAPPY CAMPING TRIP

There is nothing worse than a bad camping trip, especially since it is so easy to have a great time. To assist with making your outing a happy one, here are some pointers:

- Reserve your site ahead of time, especially if it's a weekend, a holiday, or if the campground is wildly popular. Many prime campgrounds require at least a six-month lead time on reservations. Check before you go.

- Pick your camping buddies wisely. A family trip is pretty straightforward, but you may want to reconsider including grumpy Uncle Fred who does not like bugs, sunshine, or marshmallows. After you know who is going, make sure that everyone is on the same page regarding expectations of difficulty, sleeping arrangements, and food requirements.

- Don't duplicate equipment, such as cooking pots and lanterns, among campers in your party. Carry what you need to have a good time, but don't turn the trip into a major moving experience.

- Dress appropriately for the season. Educate yourself on the high and low temperatures of the specific area you plan to visit. It may be warm at night in the summer in your backyard, but up in the mountains it will be quite chilly.

- Pitch your tent on a level surface, preferably one that is covered with leaves, pine straw, or grass. Pitch your tent on a tarp or specially designed footprint to thwart ground moisture and to protect the tent floor. Do a little site maintenance beforehand, such as picking up small rocks and sticks that can damage your tent floor and make sleep uncomfortable. If you have a separate tent rain fly but don't need it, keep it rolled up at the base of the tent in case it starts raining at midnight.

- If you are not used to sleeping on the ground, take a sleeping pad with you. Take one that is full-length and thicker than you think you might need. This will not only keep your hips from aching on hard ground, but will also help keep you warm.

- If you are not hiking in to a primitive campsite, there is no real need to skimp on food due to its weight. Plan tasty meals and bring everything you will need to prepare, cook, eat, and clean up the mess.

- If you're prone to using the bathroom multiple times at night, you should plan ahead. Leaving a warm sleeping bag and stumbling around in the dark to find the restroom, whether it be an outhouse, a fully plumbed facility, or just the woods, is second best. Keep a flashlight and any other accoutrements you may need by the tent door and know exactly where to head in the dark.

- Standing dead trees and storm-damaged living trees can pose a real hazard to tent campers. These trees may have loose or broken limbs that could fall at any time. When choosing a spot to rest or a backcountry campsite, look up.

:: CAMPING ETIQUETTE

Camping experiences can vary wildly depending on a variety of factors, such as weather, preparedness, fellow campers, and time of year. Here are a few tips on how to create good vibes with fellow campers and wildlife you encounter.

- Obtain all permits and authorization as required. Make sure you check in, pay your fee, and mark your site as directed. Don't make the mistake of grabbing a seemingly empty site that looks more appealing than yours. It could be reserved. If you are unhappy with the site you've selected, check with the campground host for other options.

- Leave only footprints. Be sensitive to the ground beneath you. Be sure to place all garbage in designated receptacles or pack it out if none are available. No one likes to see the trash someone else has left behind.

- Never spook animals. It's common for animals to wander through campsites where they may be accustomed to the presence of humans (and our food). An unannounced approach, a sudden movement, or a loud noise startles most animals. A surprised animal can be dangerous to you, to others, and to themselves. Give them plenty of space.

- Plan ahead. Know your equipment, your ability, and the area in which you are camping—and prepare accordingly. Be self-sufficient at all times; carry necessary supplies for changes in weather or other conditions. A well-executed trip is a satisfaction to you and to others.

- Be courteous to other campers, hikers, bikers, and others you encounter. If you run into the owner of a large RV, don't panic. Just wave, feign eye contact, and then walk away slowly.

- Strictly follow the campground's rules regarding the building of fires. Never burn trash. Trash smoke smells horrible, and trash debris in a fire pit or grill is unsightly.

:: VENTURING AWAY FROM THE CAMPGROUND

If you go for a hike, bike, or other excursion into the boondocks, here are some tips:

- Always carry food and water whether you are planning to go overnight or not. Food will give you energy, help keep you warm, and sustain you in an emergency situation until help arrives. You never know if you will have a stream nearby when you become thirsty. Bring potable water or treat water before drinking it from a stream. Boil or filter all found water before drinking it.

- Stay on designated trails. Most hikers get lost when they leave the path. Even on the most clearly marked trails, there is usually a point where you have to stop and consider which direction to head. If you become disoriented, don't panic. As soon as you think you may be off-track, stop, assess your current direction, and then retrace your steps back to the point where you went awry. If you become absolutely unsure of how to continue, return to your vehicle the way you came in. Should you become completely lost and have no idea of how to return to the trailhead, remaining in place along the trail and waiting for help is most often the best option for adults and always the best option for children.

- Be especially careful when crossing streams. Whether you are fording the stream or crossing on a log, make every step count. If you have any doubt about maintaining your balance on a foot log, go ahead and ford the stream instead. When fording a stream, use a trekking pole or stout stick for balance and face upstream as you cross. If a stream seems too deep to ford, turn back. Whatever is on the other side is not worth risking your life for.

- Be careful at overlooks. While these areas may provide spectacular views, they are potentially hazardous. Stay back from the edge of outcrops and be absolutely sure of your footing; a misstep can mean a nasty and possibly fatal fall.

- Know the symptoms of hypothermia. Shivering and forgetfulness are the two most common indicators of this potential killer. Hypothermia can occur at any elevation, even in the summer, especially when the hiker is wearing lightweight cotton clothing. If symptoms arise, get the victim shelter, hot liquids, and dry clothes or a dry sleeping bag.

- Take along your brain. A cool, calculating mind is the single most important piece of equipment you'll ever need on the trail. Think before you act. Watch your step. Plan ahead. Avoiding accidents before they happen is the best recipe for a rewarding and relaxing hike. Even better were my fellow tent campers, who were eager to share their knowledge about their favorite spots. They already know what beauty lies on the horizon. As this state becomes more populated, these lands become that much more precious. Enjoy them, protect them, and use them wisely.

Northwest Georgia

1

Cloudland Canyon
State Park Campground

Development on Lookout Mountain means top-notch camping and scenic overlooks.

Cloudland Canyon is an example of a state stepping in to preserve a special slice of nature for all of us to enjoy. Sure, Cloudland Canyon is developed to a degree, but part of that development consists of three campgrounds, including a delightful one for tents only. The facilities augment the natural state of things on Lookout Mountain, where Sitton Gulch Creek has carved a gorge on the mountain's western edge, allowing vistas from the rim of the gorge into the lands below.

Atop Lookout Mountain, the waters of Daniel Creek and Bear Creek cut their own gorges into the land before converging to form Sitton Gulch Creek. It is between these two creeks that the East Rim Campground lies. East Rim has 24 campsites spread along a loop meandering through the second growth, pine-oak forest commonly found on the mountaintop. Many of the sites have drive-through parking areas. That means RVs. All sites have water and

electrical hookups. A bathhouse with hot showers centers the loop. Many of the park's developed amenities are nearby. This campground may be appropriate for families with young children.

The West Rim Campground is located across Daniel Creek, away from the main section of the park. The mixed forest there is fairly thick, with second-growth trees competing with each other on a slight slope. The 48 spacious sites are spread along two loops. An understory of young hardwoods provides plenty of privacy between sites, each of which offers water and electrical hookups. Each loop has a comfort station with flush toilets and hot showers.

The Walk-In Campground is by far the best. Why? First, it allows tents only. Second, it is farthest from the rest of the park developments. Third, it is well laid out in a handsome, forested setting. Park your vehicle in the Walk-In Campground parking area. The sites are spread along a looping footpath on gently rolling terrain. The farthest sites are three-fourths of a mile from the parking area—and are worth every step.

Each site is set off in the woods, providing maximum privacy. There is ample room to spread out your gear. A short trail bisects the campground to access the comfort station, with its hot showers and flush toilets. The atmosphere is of camping in the woods,

:: Ratings

BEAUTY: ★ ★ ★ ★
PRIVACY: ★ ★ ★ ★
SPACIOUSNESS: ★ ★ ★ ★
QUIET: ★ ★ ★
SECURITY: ★ ★ ★ ★ ★
CLEANLINESS: ★ ★ ★ ★

:: Key Information

ADDRESS: 122 Cloudland Canyon Park Rd., Rising Fawn, GA 30738

OPERATED BY: Georgia State Parks

CONTACT: 706-657-4050, **gastateparks.org**

OPEN: Year-round

SITES: 30 walk-in, tents only; 73 tent and trailer; 11 backcountry

SITE AMENITIES: Picnic table, tent pad, fire ring; tent and trailer sites have electricity and water hookups

ASSIGNMENT: May choose preferred site if available

REGISTRATION: Reservations required; call 800-864-7275 at least 2 days prior to arrival; persons without reservations are guaranteed a maximum 1-night stay

FACILITIES: Water, hot showers, flush toilets, phone

PARKING: At campsites only

FEE: $16–20 walk-in sites, $25–30 tent and trailer sites, $6–8 per person backcountry sites

ELEVATION: 1,800 feet

RESTRICTIONS
■ **Pets:** On 6-foot or shorter leash
■ **Fires:** In fire rings only
■ **Alcohol:** Not allowed
■ **Vehicles:** None
■ **Other:** 14-day stay limit

not of being in a campground with a few trees around.

Cloudland Canyon would not be a state park if it didn't have natural beauty to begin with. Our visit here was particularly scenic. Fall had reached Lookout Mountain. Colorful maples and oaks mingled with the pine trees. The air was brisk. The skies were clear. We knew the views would be inspiring. We set out on the 4.8-mile West Rim Loop Trail, crossing Daniel Creek and skirting the rim of the Daniel Creek Gorge. The trail continued along the main gorge, where overlooks afforded views into the three canyons formed by Daniel Creek, Bear Creek, and Sitton Gulch Creek. We could see the point where the three gorges met, with a blaze of fall color crowning the rim.

The views continued. Below, we could see the town of Trenton. The trail left the canyon rim beyond the last overlook and reentered the mountaintop wood. Eventually, we came to the side trail that accesses the Walk-In Campground; we returned to our camp for a hot cup of coffee. Later, we took the short trail to the park's three waterfalls along Daniel Creek. Being autumn, the creek was low on water, yet we enjoyed our walk just the same.

There is still another trail: the Backcountry Loop. It follows Bear Creek and the east rim. You must find your own overlooks, so be careful. The trail requires crossing a footbridge that is often out from flooding. Inquire at the park office for the status of this trail.

Alternative activities include tennis and swimming. Lighted courts are available for day or evening use, and the pool is open from Memorial Day to Labor Day. Children will enjoy the park's playground.

Still, this is primarily a nature lover's place. And at Cloudland Canyon State Park, there is plenty to love.

1 Cloudland Canyon State Park Campground

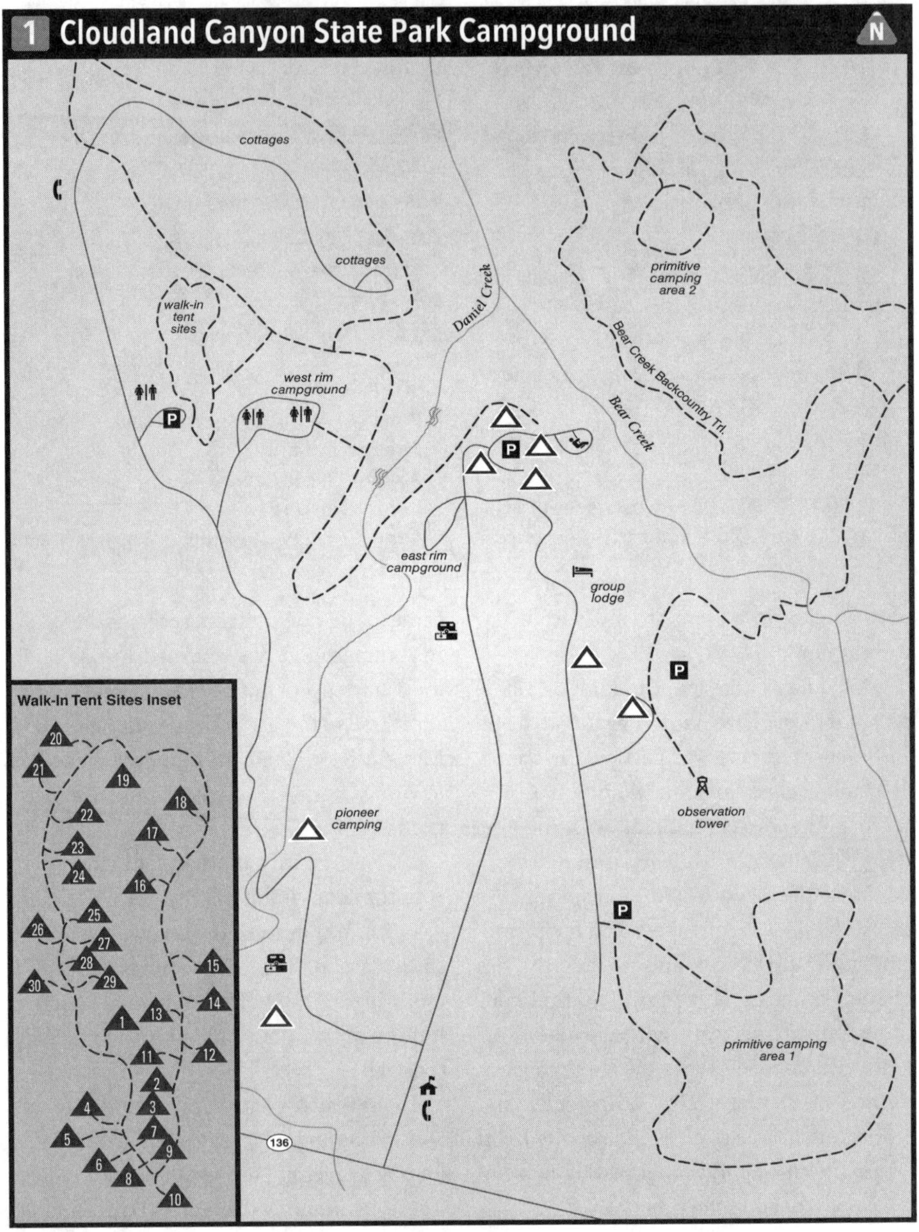

N

cottages

cottages

walk-in
tent
sites

west rim
campground

Daniel Creek

primitive
camping
area 2

Bear Creek Backcountry Trl.

Bear Creek

P

east rim
campground

group
lodge

P

observation
tower

pioneer
camping

P

primitive camping
area 1

136

Walk-In Tent Sites Inset

20
21
19
18
22
17
23
16
24
25
26
27
28   15
29
30   14
1   13
11   12
2
4   3
5   7
6   9
8
10

:: Getting There

From Trenton and I-59, take GA 136 8 miles up to Lookout Mountain. Cloudland
Canyon will be on the left.

GPS COORDINATES   N34° 49' 59.09"   W85° 28' 53.13"

Fort Mountain State Park Campground

The mysterious rock wall atop Fort Mountain is just one reason to explore one of Georgia's finest state parks.

Fort Mountain is the site of an unexplained mystery. A strange, serpentine rock wall sits atop the mountain, bounded on both sides by sheer cliffs. The wall, ranging from 2 to 6 feet in height, spans 855 feet and is broken with circular pits at 30-foot intervals, hence the name Fort Mountain. No one is sure who built it, or for what purpose, but it is speculated that the wall was some kind of fortification or was somehow related to religious activities. Either way, it is listed in the National Register of Historic Places. Later, thanks to the land donation of Ivan Allen in 1929, far-sighted Georgians also recognized the natural beauty of the area and established a state park.

Surrounded on all sides by the Chattahoochee National Forest, Fort Mountain State Park has two splendid family campgrounds that offer a variety of campsites. Set in a hardwood forest on a rolling mountainside, there are 70 shady RV/tent sites, each with water and electricity. For the more primitive tent camper, two walk-in tent areas are available. In addition, six walk-in "squirrel's nests" offer platform sites for tents only. This campground has a lot of restrictions with regard to RV size for certain campsites, but unless you plan to disregard them, they will work in your favor. If you have any questions, call ahead; reservations are strongly recommended.

Fort Mountain State Park is peaceful and safe. Quiet hours are strictly enforced. The park gates are locked between 10 p.m. and 7 a.m. The park office is staffed from 8 a.m. to 5 p.m. by accommodating park personnel. Three coin laundries provide campers with convenience. Get supplies in Chatsworth before you drive up the mountain, as there are no nearby stores in the high country.

You'll find plenty to do without ever leaving the park. A 17-acre, spring-fed lake offers fishing and a swimmer's beach complete with bathhouse. Tool around the lake in pedal boats or fishing boats, which are available for rent. For the kids, there is a playground and miniature golf course. Scheduled programs, presented by a park naturalist, are offered Wednesday through Sunday during the summer.

Naturally, Fort Mountain has trails. Near the campground, the 1.2-mile Lake Trail loops the lake. Nearby, the Big Rock Nature

:: Ratings

BEAUTY: ★ ★ ★ ★
PRIVACY: ★ ★ ★
SPACIOUSNESS: ★ ★ ★
QUIET: ★ ★ ★ ★
SECURITY: ★ ★ ★ ★ ★
CLEANLINESS: ★ ★ ★ ★ ★

:: Key Information

ADDRESS: 181 Fort Mountain Park Rd., Chatsworth, GA 30705

OPERATED BY: Georgia State Parks

CONTACT: 706-695-2621; **gastateparks.org**

OPEN: Year-round

SITES: 70 water and electric sites, 10 walk-in tent sites, 6 platform tent sites

SITE AMENITIES: Water, electrical hookups, picnic table, lantern post, cable TV hookup; walk-in tent sites have picnic table, fire ring, and water

ASSIGNMENT: By reservation or first come, first served

REGISTRATION: Reservations required; call 800-864-7275 at least 2 days prior to arrival

FACILITIES: Water, hot showers, flush toilets

PARKING: At campsites only

FEE: $26–29, $15 walk-in sites with water only, $15 platform sites

ELEVATION: 2,800 feet

RESTRICTIONS
- **Pets:** On 6-foot or shorter leash
- **Fires:** In fire rings only
- **Alcohol:** Not allowed in public areas
- **Vehicles:** Maximum 2 vehicles per site

Trail offers a cliff-edge view of the mountain, halfway along its half-mile loop. Beyond the park office is the 1.8-mile Old Fort Trail, which leads to the 855-foot-long stone wall.

Was the wall a religious site or a defensive barrier to ward off neighboring tribes? Currently, many embrace the wall's possible religious significance.

The wall runs east–west, and many speculate that an unknown tribe of sun-worshiping Native Americans built it. But Cherokee legend points to the wall being erected by a group of light-skinned, "moon-eyed people" who could see in the dark. The "moon-eyed people" may have been led by the Welsh explorer Madoc, who supposedly came north from Mobile Bay in the 14th century. Or was it built by Hernando de Soto as a defense against Native American attacks while he searched for silver and gold? Or was it something else altogether? Explore the wall and decide for yourself.

Take the side trail to the 60-year-old lookout tower, built from natural materials during the Great Depression, then refurbished in the 1970s. The mountains of northern Georgia and eastern Tennessee stand out on the horizon. Hike to the overlook deck west of the stone tower and you will see just how far it is down to the Conasauga River valley below. The really adventurous can attempt the 8.2-mile loop trail that encircles the campground. With such a high-quality campground situated amid spring wildflowers, summer's lush greenery, fall colors, and winter's crisp clarity, it's no mystery that Fort Mountain State Park is a year-round attraction.

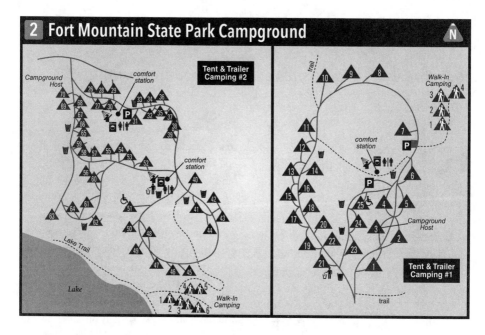

:: Getting There

From Chatsworth turn east on GA 52. Drive 7 miles up into the Cohutta Range. Fort Mountain State Park will be on your left.

GPS COORDINATES   N34° 45' 34.88"   W84° 41' 35.84"

3

Harris Branch Campground

Ridgetop walk-in tent sites overlook mountain-rimmed Carters Lake.

Harris Branch is one of the more primitive camper offerings at Carters Lake, located in the North Georgia Mountains, near Ellijay. Its nonelectric ridgetop drive-up sites, along with walk-in tent sites, make it a great destination for tent campers. Usually a primitive campground this small goes without an attendant, but not here. Harris Branch has a campground host to keep things running safely and smoothly. You will want to come here, as Carters Lake is undoubtedly a scenic Peach State destination. The lake project is run by the U.S. Army Corps of Engineers—nothing unusual about that. What is unusual is the shoreline of Carters Lake. The entire shoreline is under corps control, which means no houses, no marinas, just a wooded, serene, development-free shoreline. Steep hills and valleys, twisting arms and coves characterize this quiet impoundment.

It's a winding ride to enter Harris Branch, with its entrance station and campground host conveniently located for your arrival. The main road splits—to the right is the day-use swim beach. To the left, the campground

:: Ratings

BEAUTY: ★ ★ ★
PRIVACY: ★ ★ ★ ★
SPACIOUSNESS: ★ ★
QUIET: ★ ★ ★
SECURITY: ★ ★ ★ ★ ★
CLEANLINESS: ★ ★ ★ ★

road passes a comfort station with hot showers, then reaches the first drive-up sites, set atop a wooded ridge that drops seemingly vertically to the lake. Worry not, for the sites themselves have been leveled and bordered with landscaping timbers. Each site has gravel auto pull-ins. Maple, dogwood, oak, tulip trees, as well as pines, shade the setting. Site 1 is adequate in size and to the left of the road. Site 2 is closest to the bathhouse and has a lake view partially obscured by the trees. Note that the lake is well below the campsites and is not accessible. Sites 3 and 4 are across from one another. Site 5 is nearest the group camp area, which has a picnic shelter. Site 6 has the most privacy of the drive-up sites. A hiking trail, which leads to the recreation area swim beach, is near site 6.

The campground road curves to a loop. The walk-in tent parking area is at the far end of the loop. A trail leads to the campsites, spread on a descending peninsula. Site 7 is closest to the parking area. It too has been leveled. Views of the lake open on both sides of the ridge. Continue downhill to reach site 8. It is farther down the narrow reach of land. You will begin to see the only downside of these walk-in tent sites—to reach the lower sites, you have to practically walk through the sites closest the parking area. Site 9 is closer to the lake. Site 10 is the most coveted of all, as it is close to the lake, and just a short walk to reach water. Campers here may launch their boat from nearby and boat to this campsite. Speaking of that, Doll Mountain

:: Key Information

ADDRESS: Carters Lake Office, P.O. Box 96, Oakman, GA 30732-0096

OPERATED BY: U.S. Army Corps of Engineers

CONTACT: 706-276-4545, **www.sam .usace.army.mil/Missions/CivilWorks /Recreation/CartersLake/Camping**

OPEN: Early May–early September

SITES: 6 drive-up sites, 4 walk-in tent sites

SITE AMENITIES: Picnic table, fire ring, upright grill, lantern post

ASSIGNMENT: First come, first served

REGISTRATION: At campground entrance station

FACILITIES: Hot showers, flush toilets, coin laundry, soda machine

PARKING: At campsites and walk-in parking area

FEE: $16

ELEVATION: 1,200 feet

RESTRICTIONS
- **Pets:** On leash only
- **Fires:** In fire rings only
- **Alcohol:** At campsites only
- **Vehicles:** 2 vehicles per site
- **Other:** 14-day stay limit

Campground, very nearby, has a boat ramp. Furthermore, since Harris Branch has only 10 nonreservable campsites, you can have a backup plan of going to camp at Doll Mountain. It is also located on a steep and long peninsula running into Carters Lake, combining the rugged terrain of the landscape with the watery opportunities of the lake. It has some unusual sites, and many appealing walk-in tent sites, both far above the water and some a little closer to the water. It has 14 walk-in tent sites, 13 drive-up tent sites, and 38 water and electric sites. Doll Mountain is located three miles farther on GA 382 east beyond Harris Branch.

As mentioned, Harris Branch has a designated swim beach. You can walk the trail or drive to it, or maybe even swim to it from the walk-in tent sites! The area is cordoned off with floating buoys, and from the water rises white sand with great lake views. Above the beach, a level tier makes for a good kid watching spot, but bring your sun shade. Above that, shaded picnic tables abut the swim beach parking area. The beach is favored by campers and day users. A restroom and drink machine are located near the beach. Be apprised there is no official boat launch, but hand carried nonmotorized craft like canoes and kayaks could be put in the water by the swim beach. Whether it's on the beach or by boat, you will want to see the scenic shoreline that is Carters Lake.

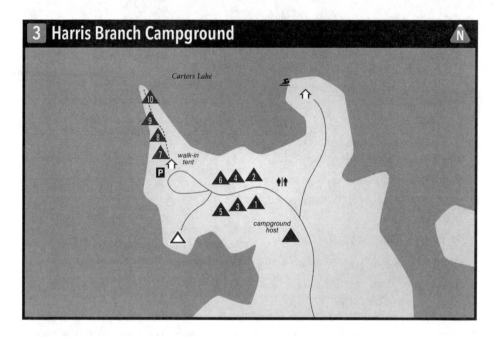

:: Getting There

From the junction of GA 53 and GA 515 near Jasper, keep north on GA 515 5.1 miles to reach GA 136. Follow GA 136 west 9.1 miles to reach GA 382 east. Turn right on GA 382 east and follow it 0.4 miles to Harris Branch Road. Turn left on Harris Branch Road and follow it 1.5 miles to dead-end into the campground.

GPS COORDINATES   N34° 36' 8.18"   W84° 37' 29.06"

4

Hickey Gap Campground

This longtime camping area along a mountain stream is free.

The Chattahoochee National Forest was established in the 1930s. Mill Creek is located on the western edge of a massive block of forestland not too far from the town of Chatsworth. Local residents began exploring the forest. A flat stretch of land along Mill Creek below Hickey Gap became a favored camping area for these locals. Eventually, the Forest Service decided to improve the flat area and establish an official campground. Today, we have an improved traditional camping area enjoyed not only by locals but also by recreation lovers from Atlanta and beyond. And it's free!

It is easy to see why this spot has attracted campers over the years. Mill Creek flows clear and clean through a level wooded area. Tall trees shade the stream, generally 8 to 10 feet in width, and maple, hickory, oak, and other hardwoods are scattered along the stream. The campground access road drops steeply from Hickey Gap to reach this flat. A short gravel road leads to site 1, which is

on the lowest part of the stream. Boulders delineate the campsite and add a rocky touch to the natural outcrops in the area. A large hill backs up to the site. Mill Creek is just steps away and makes an alluring audio accompaniment to the woodsy scenery. Site 2 is also streamside. Landscaping timbers level this site (and all the others), not just where you put your tent but also where the picnic table sits.

Site 3 is a pull-through site. The area closest to the stream is shaded, but much of the site is open to the sky overhead. The campground restrooms are directly across the gravel campground road from this site. Site 4 is farthest from the water and is the only site not directly creekside. It is heavily shaded, however. Site 5 is my favorite. It is located at the head of the flat, banked against a hill on one side and Mill Creek on the other. It is also farthest from the other campsites. The only potential downside to the site is its proximity to the unmarked trail leading upstream along Mill Creek to Mill Creek Falls. For anyone staying in site 5, the closeness of the trail makes for instant hiking, but others hiking the trail will have to almost walk through your campsite to get started or skirt around you on the hill. The gravel roads loop around beyond site 5.

A vault toilet serves the small camping area. That is the only amenity. Bring your

:: Ratings

BEAUTY: ★ ★ ★
PRIVACY: ★ ★ ★
SPACIOUSNESS: ★ ★ ★ ★
QUIET: ★ ★ ★
SECURITY: ★ ★ ★
CLEANLINESS: ★ ★ ★

:: Key Information

ADDRESS: Cohutta-Armuchee District Office, 401 G. I. Maddox Parkway, Chatsworth, GA 30705

OPERATED BY: U.S. Forest Service

CONTACT: 706-695-6736, www.fs.usda.gov/conf

OPEN: Year-round

SITES: 5

SITE AMENITIES: Picnic table, fire grate, tent pad, lantern post

ASSIGNMENT: First come, first served

REGISTRATION: Self-registration on-site

FACILITIES: Vault toilet; bring your own water.

PARKING: At campsites only

FEE: None

ELEVATION: 1,775 feet

RESTRICTIONS
- **Pets:** On leash only
- **Fires:** In fire rings only
- **Alcohol:** At campsites only
- **Vehicles:** 2 vehicles per site
- **Other:** 14-day stay limit

own water or filter it from Mill Creek. This campground can fill on nice weekends when the weather warms. Get here on Friday and you should get a campsite at that time. Otherwise, campsites are available during the week and anytime during the off-season.

You would think that if the Forest Service turned Hickey Gap into an official campground, they would turn the path to Mill Creek Falls into an official Forest Service trail. Alas, they haven't as of yet. However, that shouldn't stop you from heading along the narrow tread upstream through rich woods to reach the falls. This two-tiered drop is about 0.75 miles away. You may want to bring your fishing rod along. The Georgia Department of Natural Resources stocks this creek twice weekly during the warm season. You can follow the creek downstream as well, although no formal trail exists.

Other recreation requires leaving the campground but is no more than a few miles away. On the way in you pass the Rocky Flats ORV Trail. This path is popular with mountain bikers, as well as those on motorized

wheels. The Sumac Creek Trail, open to hikers and often used by mountain bikers, is 0.7 miles away on Forest Road 630. This path makes a long-distance 12.5-mile double loop. During the trip it drops off ridgelines to Sumac Creek three times! Hikers would be better served by keeping on FR 630 2.2 miles to the Hickory Creek trailhead, which leads into the Cohutta Wilderness. I have hiked every trail in the Cohutta Wilderness and proclaim it to be one of Georgia's outstanding natural jewels. Wooded ridges, clear mountain streams, and nature on nature's terms awaits. The Hickory Creek Trail will take you down from on high to Rough Creek, which you follow to its confluence with the Conasauga River at Bray Field. No matter whether you go upstream or downstream on the Conasauga, the riverside scenery will not disappoint. The crystalline watercourse tumbles over boulders into pools where you can take a heat-relieving dip in nature's swimming pool, returning to your long-established campground at Hickey Gap.

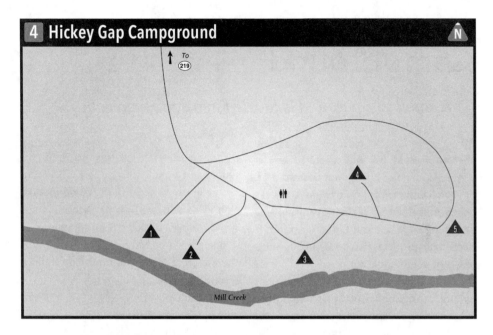

:: Getting There

From the county courthouse in Chatsworth, take US 411 North 7.2 miles to Grassy Street. Turn right here and follow it 0.4 miles over the railroad tracks to Crandall-Ellijay Road. Turn right on Crandall-Ellijay Road and follow it just a short distance to Mill Creek Road. Turn left on Mill Creek Road (FR 630), and follow it 6.5 miles to the camping area, on your right.

GPS COORDINATES   N34° 53' 40.93"   W84° 40' 5.29"

5

Jacks River Fields Campground

This small campground is located in a cool, high valley.

The Forest Service should consider renaming this campground. For starters, it is on South Fork Jacks River, not the Jacks River. And the days of this streamside area being fields are just about over. The forest is reclaiming the fields that once ran down this ridge-rimmed valley. But what's in a name? What we do have here is a small, pretty campground in a quiet nook of the Chattahoochee National Forest. Water- and land-based recreation is immediately at hand. If you like hiking long trails, two of the longest in the Southeast converge in this area.

South Fork Jacks River is born on Flat Top Mountain to the southeast. This mountain also forms the eastern flank of the valley. Pink Knob and the ridge on which it stands border the river to the west. Chilly mountain waters flow from these high ridges. The campground lies in a flat where a small, unnamed stream meets South Fork Jacks River. A ranger cabin once stood at the site. It was likely a homesite before that. Nowadays, a small gravel loop circles the campground, which still is partly open

overhead, especially in the middle of the loop. Site 1 actually sits on part of the concrete slab that was once the cabin foundation. This slab, with some additional site work, has been turned into an all-access site. A small, unnamed stream gurgles nearby in the shade of rhododendron. Curve down toward the river, passing site 2, which is partly shaded by tulip trees. Site 3 is also along the small stream.

Site 4 is the most popular campsite. It is located at the confluence of the small stream and South Fork Jacks River. Notice the peeling bark of the yellow birch trees here. Yellow birch trees grow in cool climes, in which this high valley is located. Site 5 is directly along South Fork Jacks River, which at this point is 10–12 feet wide. A beaver pond is just below the campground here. The gravel road turns away from the river, although site 6 is not far from the water. I stayed in site 7 because the white pine tree here afforded deep shade.

A dirt road leads across the unnamed stream up to a small clearing. This is the small equestrian camping area. A gravel parking area lies next to the clearing, which is broken with boulders. A tall white pine shades the clearing center. There are no campsite amenities here, but there are horse-hitching posts in the woods adjacent to the clearing. A small footbridge also connects the equestrian area to the main campground. The entire campground fills only

:: Ratings

BEAUTY: ★ ★ ★ ★
PRIVACY: ★ ★ ★
SPACIOUSNESS: ★ ★ ★ ★
QUIET: ★ ★ ★ ★
SECURITY: ★ ★ ★
CLEANLINESS: ★ ★ ★

:: Key Information

ADDRESS: Cohutta-Armuchee District Office, 401 G. I. Maddox Parkway, Chatsworth, GA 30705

OPERATED BY: U.S. Forest Service

CONTACT: 706-695-6736, www.fs.usda.gov/conf

OPEN: Year-round

SITES: 7

SITE AMENITIES: Picnic table, fire ring, tent pad, lantern post

ASSIGNMENT: First come, first served

REGISTRATION: Self-registration on-site

FACILITIES: Vault toilet

PARKING: At campsites only

FEE: $5

ELEVATION: 2,700 feet

RESTRICTIONS
- **Pets:** On leash only
- **Fires:** In fire rings only
- **Alcohol:** At campsites only
- **Vehicles:** 2 vehicles per site
- **Other:** 14-day stay limit

during summer holiday weekends. If you want some real mountain water, a spring is located just across the unnamed stream on the dirt road leading to the equestrian camping area. The rocked-in spring has a pipe for easy access. Be aware that this chilly water, likely the water source for the old ranger cabin, is untreated.

Trout fishing is popular around here. Wily brown trout ply the South Fork Jacks River, and most fishing is done downstream. The South Fork Trail starts at the road bridge crossing South Fork and heads downstream. It is only 10 minutes of walking to meet the Benton MacKaye Trail. If you take a right on the BMT, this trail goes more miles than you can walk in a day to its southern terminus atop Spring Mountain, also the terminus for the Appalachian Trail. It's only 0.6 mile to FR 22 at Dyer Gap and 2 miles to the top of 3,732-foot Flat Top Mountain, the site of an old fire tower. Or you can go downstream along South Fork Jacks River, through evergreen woods broken by more open areas (the

Benton MacKaye Trail runs in conjunction with the South Fork Trail at this point). The South Fork is never far away, slicing through gorges into deep pools and sometimes widening where old fields once were. Beavers have dammed many parts of the river. It is 1.6 miles to the point where the Benton MacKaye Trail leaves South Fork in Rich Cove.

The South Fork Trail keeps forward and soon ends at FR 126. Mountain bikers make a loop by turning right on FR 126 to reach Watson Gap, then turn right on FR 64 and follow it to Dyer Gap and down to the campground. The Pinhoti Trail, a long-distance path connecting the mountains of Alabama and Georgia, traces the nearby Mountaintown Creek Trail and will connect to South Fork Trail from the west. Call ahead at the ranger station for the latest Pinhoti information. While you're at it, order a Chattahoochee National Forest map before you come. And when you come, you will find that, despite the misleading name, it is no mistake to tent camp at Jacks River Fields.

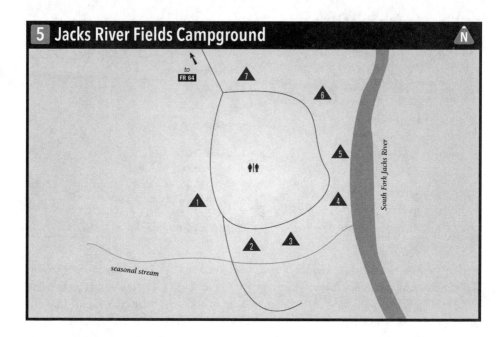

:: Getting There

From Blue Ridge, Georgia, where US 76 and GA 5 diverge, head north on US 76 3.7 miles to Old State Road 2. A sign will say "Old S. R. 2." Turn left here and follow Old State Road 2 10.6 miles to Watson Gap, located at the intersection of FR 64 and FR 22. Turn left on FR 64 and follow it 4 miles to the campground, on your left just after the bridge crossing South Fork Jacks River.

GPS COORDINATES N34° 54' 15.53" W84° 31' 18.24"

6

Lake Conasauga Campground

Camp, fish, and hike in the high country around Georgia's highest lake.

Set in the rugged highlands of the western Chattahoochee National Forest, 19-acre Lake Conasauga is a mountaintop oasis adjacent to the 34,000-acre Cohutta Wilderness, Georgia's largest wilderness area. Tent campers will be well rewarded after the long gravel drive that deters all but the most determined RVers. Expect a nearly full campground on weekends. Make sure to bring everything you need—civilization is far away. After you go boating, hiking, swimming, fishing, and wildlife viewing, you will be ready to kick back in the breezy campground.

The campground is located near the lake and divided into three areas. The main campground has 31 sites divided into two loops. The upper loop is on a forested ridge with 12 spacious and private sites. It has several water spigots and a central bathroom atop the ridge with flush toilets for each gender. The lakeside lower loop is shaded by white pine with little understory. Five sites are actually lakefront. Those and the other sites offer an appealing view of the clear blue waters ringed by rhododendrons. A comfort station and water spigot are located at the head of the loop.

The second loop area holds only four sites in a grassy clearing ringed with trees, but they have no view of the lake. However, the Lakeshore Trail makes the lake instantly accessible. Flush toilets and water are nearby. This small area has an isolated feel to it.

The final five sites sit in the overflow area atop the ridge above the lake. The area has flush toilets but no water, though a short trip to the other loops can amend that problem. The breezes are stronger here, and the area has a mountaintop feel to it. A campground host is located at the largest loop on summer weekends. Recycling stations are located in each camping area.

If you're finding it hard to pick a site, you will really be hard-pressed to decide what to do first. To explore Lake Conasauga, dammed in 1940 by the Civilian Conservation Corps (CCC), you can take the 0.8-mile Lakeshore Trail that courses through trees and bushes along the water's edge. A grassy glade with benches covers the dam. Sit down, relax, and absorb the atmosphere. Or use a canoe or small johnboat and fish for bream, bass, or trout. Only electric motors are allowed. Want to take a dip? Across the lake from the campground is a ringed-off

:: Ratings

BEAUTY: ★ ★ ★ ★ ★
PRIVACY: ★ ★ ★ ★
SPACIOUSNESS: ★ ★ ★ ★
QUIET: ★ ★ ★ ★
SECURITY: ★ ★ ★ ★
CLEANLINESS: ★ ★ ★ ★

:: Key Information

ADDRESS: Cohutta-Armuchee District Office, 401 G. I. Maddox Parkway, Chatsworth, GA 30705	**REGISTRATION:** Self-registration on-site
	FACILITIES: Water spigots, flush toilets
OPERATED BY: U.S. Forest Service	**PARKING:** At campsites only
CONTACT: 706-695-6736, www.fs.usda.gov/conf	**FEE:** $10
	ELEVATION: 3,150 feet
OPEN: Mid-April–October	**RESTRICTIONS**
SITES: 35, including overflow sites	■ **Pets:** On leash only
SITE AMENITIES: Fire ring, picnic table, lantern post, tent pad	■ **Fires:** In fire rings only
	■ **Alcohol:** At campsites only
ASSIGNMENT: First come, first served	■ **Vehicles:** 22-foot trailer length limit
	■ **Other:** 14-day stay limit

swimming beach. You can reach it from the picnic area or the Lakeshore Trail.

Start hiking right from your campsite. The Songbird and Grassy Mountain Trails are instantly accessible. Wildlife viewing is made easy by the 0.6-mile Songbird Trail. The Forest Service has cleared small plots along the trail to make a better habitat for the owl, woodcock, and kingfisher that live here. Beavers have dammed the trailside stream, strengthening biodiversity with their ponds that provide a habitat for numerous amphibians. The 2-mile Grassy Mountain Tower Trail climbs gradually to the 3,692-foot fire tower. From the tower you can see the forested Cohutta Wilderness and the Southern Appalachians as they stretch northward into Tennessee.

Just a short distance away from Lake Conasauga are forest roads that circle the southern half of the Cohutta Wilderness. No fewer than six trails lead from these roads into the heart of the Cohutta. Make the most of your adventuring with a map of the wilderness, which can be obtained at the Ranger Station in Chatsworth. The Tearbritches Trail (Forest Trail 9) starts just east of the campground. It crosses Bald Mountain and then descends to Bray Field along the Conasauga River. The Conasauga River has a reputation as Georgia's cleanest, clearest waterway. Chestnut Lead Trail (FT 11) drops into the lower Conasauga in 1.8 miles. East Cowpen Trail (FT 30) traverses the high country at the heart of the wilderness. Large trees, wildlife, and good fishing are all Cohutta hallmarks.

Conasauga is an area of Georgian superlatives: the highest lake, the cleanest water, the largest wilderness. Come here with high expectations. You won't be disappointed.

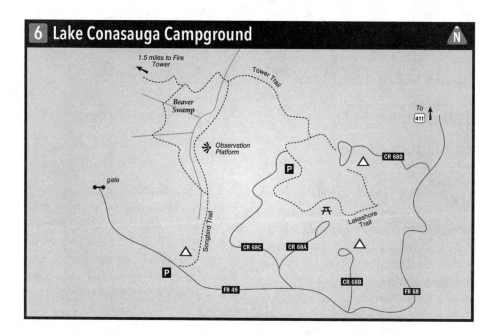

:: Getting There

From Chatsworth take US 411 North 4 miles; turn right at the traffic light in Eton. Follow FS 18 East 10 miles. Turn left on FS 68 and follow it 10 miles. Lake Conasauga will be on your right.

GPS COORDINATES   N34° 51' 36.40"   W84° 39' 6.11"

7

McKaskey Creek Campground

This campground is your best option for overnighting on Allatoona Lake.

Allatoona Lake is a large impoundment northwest of Atlanta that provides drinking water for much of the metro area. It is also a popular recreation destination for Atlantans. Despite the millions in the greater area of Georgia's capital city, there is generally enough water left over for them to fish, swim, and cool off during the summer. McKaskey Creek Campground, on a narrow arm of the lake's northwest corner, is the best destination for tent campers wishing to enjoy Lake Allatoona. It is relatively quiet and away from the hustle and bustle of larger, wider portions of Allatoona. And if you live in Atlanta, hustle and bustle is what you are trying to escape while on a tent-camping adventure.

Located on a peninsula and nearly encircled by water, this campground setup provides a maximum number of waterfront campsites. The first 6 sites, 1–6, are located on a short spur circle road shaded by tall pines with an understory of dogwood and maple. These sites exemplify the

:: Ratings

BEAUTY: ★ ★ ★
PRIVACY: ★ ★
SPACIOUSNESS: ★ ★ ★ ★
QUIET: ★ ★ ★
SECURITY: ★ ★ ★ ★ ★
CLEANLINESS: ★ ★ ★ ★ ★

good quality of corps campground sites. The large, well-built sites are two-tiered, angling toward the water. These sites are reservable and have electricity. Despite the electricity, sites 2–5 are classified as tent sites. Folks like to jump off a rock into the water near site 3.

Sites 7–9 are on the main campground road and are a little too open for the hot Georgia summer. A loop leading left has sites 10–22. These sites are large, and most have electricity. However, the three sites closest to the lake, 18–20, are electricity-free and my favorites. Each overlooks the McKaskey Creek arm of the lake. Campsite 18 has a great tent spot and steps leading to the water. Large sweet gum trees shade site 19, directly waterside. Site 20 is extra spacious and also has steps leading to the water. However, they are not reservable. The modern bathhouse is located on this loop.

Sites 23–31 are grouped together. Site 31 is adjacent to the swim beach and overlooks the water, along with 27–30. Red needles litter the ground below tall pines. Avoid sites 23–26, as they are away from the water. Sites 32 and 33 are in the middle of the action, beside the swim beach and boat ramp. Don't expect solitude or privacy here. You might as well be camping on stage at site 33. Sites 34–37 are on the main campground road and will do if all other sites are filled. Sites 38 and 39 are coveted tent sites close to the

:: Key Information

ADDRESS: P.O. Box 487, Cartersville, GA 30120-0487

OPERATED BY: Army Corps of Engineers

CONTACT: 678-721-6700, **www.sam .usace.army.mil/Missions/CivilWorks /Recreation/AllatoonaLake/Camping;** reservations 877-444-6777, **recreation.gov**

OPEN: Late March-early September

SITES: 19 nonelectric, 32 electric

SITE AMENITIES: Picnic table, fire grate, lantern post, tent pad, upright grill

ASSIGNMENT: First come, first served and by reservation

REGISTRATION: At entrance station

FACILITIES: Hot showers, flush toilets, water spigots, laundry

PARKING: At campsites only

FEE: $20 nonelectric, $26–30 electric

ELEVATION: 850 feet

RESTRICTIONS
- **Pets:** On leash only; 2-pet limit
- **Fires:** In fire rings only
- **Alcohol:** At campsites only
- **Vehicles:** 3 vehicles per site
- **Other:** 14-day stay limit

water and the boat ramp. Avoid sites 43–45. Sites 40 and 41 are very large.

Sites 46–50 are on a spur road away from the main camp. Site 46 is well shaded, but the others have just scattered shade from spindly pines. These sites overlook a tiny cove of the lake.

The Army Corps of Engineers started work on this lake in 1941, but World War II interrupted completion. The gates were closed on the dam in 1950, long before Atlanta became the boomtown it is today. The lake not only provides drinking water for Atlanta, but also reduces flooding in the lower Etowah River valley and provides power production, as well as a little water recreation at places like McKaskey Creek.

McKaskey is a well-kept, family-oriented campground, where the rules are enforced so all can have a good time. If you are looking to raise a ruckus, go elsewhere. The campground fills on summer holiday weekends and spring break weekends.

Interestingly, waterskiing is not allowed here on Saturday, Sunday, and holidays. This rule keeps the atmosphere a little quieter than on most large lakes. The McKaskey Creek arm is a bit narrow for fast boating anyway. Fishing is a definite option. A pretty little beach offers swimming opportunities directly from the campground.

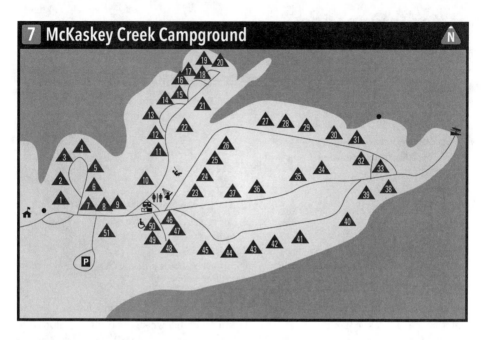

:: Getting There

From Exit 290 on I-75, take GA 20 east for 0.1 mile to GA 20 Spur. Make a quick right turn onto GA 20 Spur and follow it 1.3 miles to McKaskey Creek Road. Veer left onto McKaskey Creek Road and follow it 1 mile to dead-end into the campground.

GPS COORDINATES   N34° 11.367'   W84° 43.061'

8

The Pocket Campground

The attractive nature of the campground matches the attractive nature around the campground.

The Pocket gets its unusual name from its location. It is a large, relatively flat slice of land. There's nothing unusual about that; however, ridges surround the flat in a horseshoe shape, the flat being "The Pocket." Mill Mountain and Horn Mountain form the horseshoe. This pretty location offers "springside" camping on Pocket Creek. Year-round springs emit from the creekbed at the campground, enhancing an already attractive locale and good-quality campground. The Pocket has a little history too. The site housed Civilian Conservation Corps Camp F-16 from 1938 to 1942.

Enter the campground on a paved road with paved auto pull-ins. A campground host is on the hill to your left during the warm season. The first four sites are located along Pocket Creek, which flows to the right of the road. These sites are well maintained, as is the whole campground, but are a little too exposed because trees were removed following pine-beetle infestation.

:: Ratings

BEAUTY: ★ ★ ★ ★
PRIVACY: ★ ★ ★ ★
SPACIOUSNESS: ★ ★ ★ ★
QUIET: ★ ★ ★ ★
SECURITY: ★ ★ ★ ★
CLEANLINESS: ★ ★ ★ ★

Reach the loop portion of the campground. Pine and oak woods tower overhead. Shade is plentiful. Dogwood, beech, and maple trees enhance the lush woods with plenty of underbrush for campsite privacy. Sites 5 and 6 also back up to Pocket Creek. Pass the picnic area to your right. This is one end of the Pocket Loop Trail. It bridges Pocket Creek by a spring (concrete-lined) and passes by the day-use picnic area across the creek.

Restrooms are located just inside the campground loop. Five water spigots are located throughout the campground. More attractive sites, 9–12, resume on a spur loop. These are large and level. Two sites are directly streamside. Site 8 is inside the spur loop and is the only undesirable site in the whole campground. The main loop has more appealing sites. Site 15 is good for solitude lovers. The other end of the Pocket Loop Trail comes in near site 16. A serene spur road has five more sites, 17–21, beneath tall pines. One of these sites is a double site. The final six sites are also well cared for. Site 27 is wooded but backs up to a grassy wildlife clearing. The Pocket will fill on summer holiday weekends and nice-weather weekends in late spring and early fall. You should be able to get a site if you arrive early on a Friday, however.

The campsites are nice enough that you may not want to leave camp. However, there's a pretty world to explore in these

:: Key Information

ADDRESS: Cohutta-Armuchee District Office, 401 G. I. Maddox Parkway, Chatsworth, GA 30705	**REGISTRATION:** Self-registration on-site
	FACILITIES: Flush toilets, water spigots
OPERATED BY: U.S. Forest Service	**PARKING:** At campsites only
CONTACT: 706-695-6736, www.fs.usda.gov/conf	**FEE:** $10
	ELEVATION: 900 feet
OPEN: April–October	**RESTRICTIONS**
SITES: 27	■ **Pets:** On leash only
SITE AMENITIES: Picnic table, fire grate, tent pad, lantern post	■ **Fires:** In fire rings only
	■ **Alcohol:** Prohibited
ASSIGNMENT: First come, first served	■ **Vehicles:** 2 vehicles per site
	■ **Other:** 14-day stay limit

parts. Spring-fed Pocket Creek is just steps away. Kids can play or wade in it. Pocket Creek flows into Johns Creek, which is stocked with trout. Two all-access fishing piers are nearby, just south on Pocket Road. The Pocket Trail makes a 2.5-mile loop, crisscrossing several other springs, and seeps on the way in between finger ridges dipping down the mountainsides. The Pocket Nature Trail makes a 1-mile loop and offers interpretive signage along the way.

Keown Falls and Johns Mountain Overlook and Trail are just a short jaunt down Pocket Road. They are part of the Keown Falls Scenic Area. Keown Falls, a set of twin cascades, makes a 50-foot drop and is more impressive in spring when the water flows more strongly. The Keown Falls Trail makes a 1.7-mile loop, passing an observation deck.

You can also check out Keown Falls from the top down via the Johns Mountain Trail, which leaves from the Johns Mountain Overlook. It offers views of ridges fading into the distance and travels along a bluff line, dipping to Keown Falls before returning to the observation area on an old roadbed.

Pocket Road itself is part of the Ridge and Valley Scenic Byway, which essentially encircles Johns Mountain. The byway begins at GA 136 and GA 201, then heads south on Armuchee Road to GA 27. It then heads south on GA 27, turns left on GA 156, and turns left on Floyd Springs Road to Johns Creek Road to Pocket Road. After tooling around on this marked byway, you will have a good idea of what this part of the Chattahoochee National Forest is all about from your base camp at The Pocket.

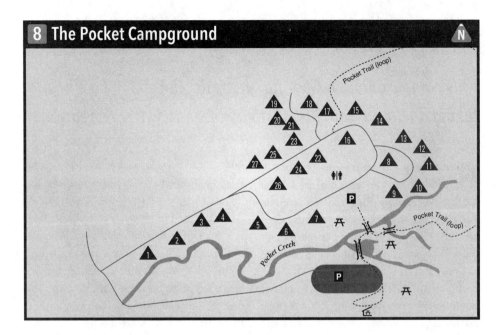

:: Getting There

From La Fayette, take GA 136 East 13.5 miles to Pocket Road, 0.5 miles east of the intersection of GA 136 and GA 201. Turn right onto Pocket Road and follow it 7 miles to the campground, on your left.

GPS COORDINATES   N34° 35' 6.70"   W85° 04' 47.01"

9

Ridgeway Campground

This campground on Georgia's least developed big lake has hiking and mountain biking, in addition to water recreation.

Ridgeway Campground is about as rustic as you can get on a big lake in Georgia. For starters, Ridgeway is located on Carters Lake, an impoundment of the Coosawattee River. The U.S. Army Corps of Engineers, who developed Carters Lake, manage not only the lake but all the shoreline surrounding it too. This means you see nothing but hillside forests rising from the shoreline, not houses and docks and marinas and such. This also means a quieter and less crowded experience on the lake and at this campground, which features nothing but walk-in tent sites high on a ridgeline. You can enjoy this land on hiking and biking trails that emanate directly from the recreation area.

The campground itself is set on the inside of a bend in the Coosawattee River arm of Carters Lake. This narrow ribbon of water, the Coosawattee arm, lies far below the actual camping area, which seems decidedly more land than lake in these parts. The recreation access road splits just before reaching the actual camping area. The road leading right heads down to the area trails and the lake

boat ramp. The road leading left traverses the height of the bend. The walk-in campsites are divided into individual sets, each with a small parking area of its own.

Reach the first two sites on a little hill to the right. These sites are well shaded by a pine, oak, and hickory woodland and are just a few steps from the parking area. The next three sites are near the campground fee station. The wooded sites require just a short walk to reach. They have an additional common fire circle. Ahead is a rib ridge emanating away from the main ridgeline. Four sites descend along the rib ridge, with the last one in a saddle. The Ridgeway Mountain Biking Trail passes this line of sites. A short path leads to the campground pump well.

The next four sites are on a small knob before the end of the road. A vault toilet for each gender lies at the end of the road. A pump well and vault toilet are also located down by the boat ramp. Reach the end of the road and the last parking area. Two sites are just to the right in a somewhat open area. The final five sites extend straight out of the ridgeline. These sites are on the level part of the ridge, which drops very steeply off on both sides. The lake is far away. A group fire circle is at the far end of these sites.

Fishing is the most popular water pastime here. The U.S. Army Corps of Engineers has a detailed information sheet on fishing at Carters Lake that would prove helpful to those vying for walleye, bass, and bream.

:: Ratings

BEAUTY: ★ ★ ★
PRIVACY: ★ ★ ★ ★
SPACIOUSNESS: ★ ★ ★
QUIET: ★ ★ ★ ★ ★
SECURITY: ★ ★ ★
CLEANLINESS: ★ ★ ★ ★

:: Key Information

ADDRESS: P.O. Box 96, Oakman, GA 30732	**ASSIGNMENT:** First come, first served
OPERATED BY: U.S. Army Corps of Engineers	**REGISTRATION:** Self-registration on-site
	FACILITIES: Vault toilet, pump well
CONTACT: 706-334-2248, **www.sam .usace.army.mil/Missions/CivilWorks /Recreation/CartersLake/Camping**	**PARKING:** At walk-in parking areas
	FEE: $10
	ELEVATION: 1,200 feet
OPEN: Year-round	**RESTRICTIONS**
SITES: 18	■ **Pets:** On leash only
	■ **Fires:** In fire rings only
SITE AMENITIES: Picnic table, fire ring, tent pad, trash can	■ **Alcohol:** At campsites only
	■ **Vehicles:** 2 vehicles per site
	■ **Other:** 14-day stay limit

The narrowness of the lake around Ridgeway dissuades recreational boating, such as waterskiing, but is ideal for slower-paced scenic boating. The Ridgeway boat ramp is just a short drive from the campground.

The best advice for those wanting to enjoy the trails here is to get a map ahead of time. The Ridgeway Mountain Bike Trail makes a 6-mile loop, encircling the campground. This single- and double-track path traverses the steep ridges divided by small creeks. In places, the trail splits into sections for more advanced mountain bikers. Short, steep climbs are sometimes followed by technical downhills. Try the Tumbling Waters Nature Trail for more of a slow-motion path on which you can more completely appreciate the beauty of the Carters Lake area. This walking trail starts near the boat ramp and soon forks. One fork heads upstream along Tails Creek to a viewing deck overlooking a cascade. The other fork travels over a bridge, then up an old tailrace from a mill that was once along Tails Creek, and ends at another observation deck on Tails Creek. This second fork also has a loop portion to vary your return. After you see how different the Carters Lake experience is, you will be returning to this northwest Georgia impoundment for more camping adventures.

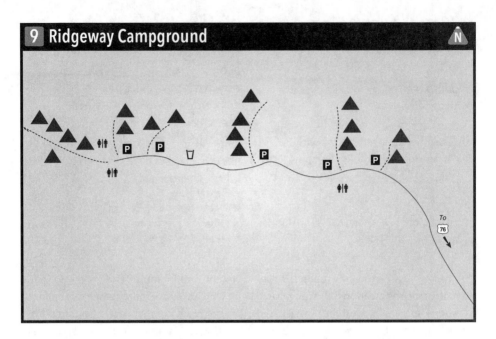

:: Getting There

From the junction of GA 515 and US 76 in East Ellijay, head west on US 76 8.7 miles to the signed turn on Gilmer County Road 54. Turn left on CR 54 and follow it 3 miles to the campground.

GPS COORDINATES   N34° 39' 10.02"   W84° 36' 4.28"

10

Sweetwater Campground

Sweetwater offers numerous lakefront tent sites on popular Allatoona Lake.

Did you know that Allatoona Lake, northwest of Atlanta, has been the most popular U.S. Army Corps of Engineers lake in the United States the past few years? For Allatoona campers, there are more than 600 campsites spread among its campgrounds. Sweetwater campground is among the largest, but it is also among the best. And it offers numerous lakefront non-electric campsites that offer a great getaway for Atlantans and other Georgians. It also provides drinking water for much of metro Atlanta, especially Cobb County, as well as Cartersville. Despite the millions in the greater area of Georgia's capital city, there is generally enough water leftover for them to fish, swim, and cool off during the summer. And Sweetwater's well-maintained lakefront sites provide the ideal venue.

The camping area is stretched along the north shore of the long lake, bordered by gently rolling piney hills, with a maximum number of waterfront sites. The corps, when building the campground, left electricity out of the sites that were lowest, which is a boon

:: Ratings

BEAUTY: ★ ★ ★ ★
PRIVACY: ★ ★
SPACIOUSNESS: ★ ★ ★ ★
QUIET: ★ ★
SECURITY: ★ ★ ★ ★ ★
CLEANLINESS: ★ ★ ★ ★

for us tent campers. Pass the campground entrance station and reach the first camping area on your left, with sites 96–149. Tall pines shade the camps, which are mostly electric. Here, in the lowest areas, which also happen to be closest to the lake, are the nonelectric sites, 116–131. They offer superlative lake views. The shade is adequate, but the pine needles and cones under the trees do nothing for campsite privacy, though the sites are well spaced from one another. A few hardwoods, such as dogwoods, are interspersed in the pines. The next good nonelectric sites are 112–115, though they are a bit close to the day-use beach, which becomes crowded on nice summer weekends. Another set of sites, 96–103, is also nonelectric and looks out on a creek flowing into the lake, and the lake itself. Campsite 103 would be good for kids, as it borders the day-use area, which not only has a camper's beach but also a playground.

Sites 78–95 also face the lake but are open to the sun overhead. Bring a sun shelter when staying here. The lowest ones are nonelectric. The paved campground road continues to another piney area by the boat ramp. I highly recommend sites 70–75. They are shaded, well spaced, and overlook the lake. And the campground goes on, into a hillier area with many hardwoods to go with the pines. More lakefront campsites continue. Pass the group camp, located on a hill. You will think you have entered a different campground. Wooded and secluded sites,

:: Key Information

ADDRESS: U.S. Army Corps of Engineers, Allatoona Lake Office, P.O. Box 487, Cartersville, GA 30120-0487

OPERATED BY: U.S. Army Corps of Engineers

CONTACT: 678-721-6700, **www.sam .usace.army.mil/Missions/CivilWorks /Recreation/AllatoonaLake/Camping;** reservations 877-444-6777, **recreation.gov**

OPEN: Late March–early September

SITES: 41 nonelectric, 105 electric

SITE AMENITIES: Picnic table, fire ring, upright grill, lantern post, tent pad, most also have spigots

ASSIGNMENT: By reservation and first come, first served

REGISTRATION: At campground entrance station

FACILITIES: Hot showers, flush toilets, laundry

PARKING: At campsites only

FEE: $20 nonelectric sites, $26–30 electric sites

ELEVATION: 840 feet

RESTRICTIONS
■ **Pets:** On leash only
■ **Fires:** In fire rings only
■ **Alcohol:** At campsites only
■ **Vehicles:** 3 vehicles per site
■ **Other:** 14-day stay limit

1–27, are cut into steep hillsides. Though these sites have electricity, they have short paved pull-ins, with the picnic table and other amenities set on leveled areas on the hillside, effectively eliminating RVs, except at the pull-through sites. Most have lake views, yet they have enough woods around them to give adequate privacy.

When reserving a campsite here, ask for a nonelectric waterfront site and you will do well. If privacy is an issue, seek sites 1–27. I do recommend reservations, as this campground can fill on summer weekends, especially holidays.

Campers like to enjoy the lake, from skiing to swimming to sunbathing. Kids and adults like to pedal the roads here on

their bikes. It's a big, fun place that offers a group experience on a busy lake. The rules are enforced so all can have a good time. If you are looking to raise a ruckus, go elsewhere.

The U.S. Army Corps of Engineers started work on this lake in 1941, but World War II interrupted completion. The gates were closed on the dam in 1950, long before Atlanta became the boomtown it is today. The lake not only provides drinking water for Atlanta, but also reduces flooding on the lower Etowah River valley and provides power production, as well as a little water recreation at places like Sweetwater Campground. Just remember, don't pee in the water because you may be drinking it later.

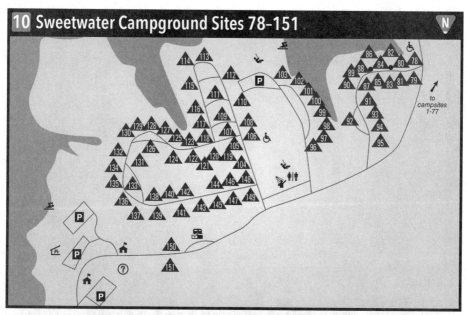

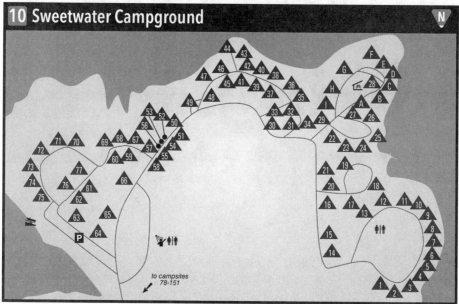

:: Getting There

From Exit 390 on I-75, take GA 20 east 10.6 miles to Fields Chapel Road. Turn right on Fields Chapel Road and follow it 1.4 miles to dead-end at the campground.

GPS COORDINATES   N34° 11' 46.48"   W84° 34' 40.21"

Northeast Georgia

11

Amicalola Falls State Park Campground

This mountain state park has the highest waterfall in the East.

The word Amicalola is Cherokee for "tumbling waters." This state park features a 729-foot waterfall, Amicalola Falls, reputed to be the tallest fall in the East. Yet this state park is much more than a waterfall. Overlain on a scenic mountainscape, the park offers an intimate campground, first-rate hiking trails, some of the best interpretive programs anywhere in the country, and a lodge where you can stuff yourself silly after your outdoorsy adventures. One more word about the trails here: Included among them is the approach trail to the master path of the East, the Appalachian Trail, where it begins atop nearby Springer Mountain. Hikers intent on hiking the AT all the way from Springer Mountain to Mount Katahdin in Maine, a six-month endeavor, often spend some time here at Amicalola Falls State Park. Although your stay here will be much shorter, it can certainly be as rewarding.

The campground was made "campable" with a surprising amount of leveling work using landscaping timbers. You will find the

:: Ratings

BEAUTY: ★ ★ ★
PRIVACY: ★ ★ ★
SPACIOUSNESS: ★ ★ ★
QUIET: ★ ★ ★ ★
SECURITY: ★ ★ ★ ★ ★
CLEANLINESS: ★ ★ ★ ★

campground located on a dry, wooded slope not far from Amicalola Falls. The drive to the campground from the park office is surprisingly steep, and the cooler temperatures up here reveal this elevation gain.

Pass campsite 1 before reaching the loop part of the campground. Turn right, passing the campground host. Ahead is the bathhouse. Larger sites lie on the lower outside edge of the loop. Curve up a hill past campsite 11. Some of the most reworked sites are on the inside of the loop here. Dip to a low point, then climb again to complete the small camping circle. Being small is one of the most appealing aspects of this campground. The park could easily fill two or three times the sites, but keeping it small stays in tune with the rustic atmosphere of this park, which is nearly encircled by the vast Chattahoochee National Forest. Be aware that this small number of sites comes at a price: The campground will fill nearly every weekend between late March and early November. During the week, it can be fairly busy when the weather is nice. Reserve a site and show up early to claim a good spot (you can reserve a site for a given night but not a specific site for a given night).

Checking out Amicalola Falls is a must. It's a short jaunt to the overlook atop the falls. This view allows a good look to the south and east, but to appreciate the falls you must take the Base of Falls Trail, which

:: Key Information

ADDRESS: 240 Amicalola Falls State Park Rd., Dawsonville, GA 30534	**FACILITIES:** Hot showers, flush toilets, laundry
OPERATED BY: Georgia State Parks	**PARKING:** At campsites only
CONTACT: 706-265-4703, **gastateparks .org;** reservations 800-573-9656	**FEE:** $25 tent; $28 RV
OPEN: Year-round	**ELEVATION:** 2,600 feet
SITES: 25	**RESTRICTIONS**
SITE AMENITIES: Picnic table, fire grate, lantern post, tent pad, water, electricity	■ **Pets:** On leash only
	■ **Fires:** In fire rings only
ASSIGNMENT: First come, first served or by reservation	■ **Alcohol:** At campsites only
	■ **Vehicles:** 2 vehicles per site
REGISTRATION: At park lodge	■ **Other:** 14-day stay limit

leads 0.3 miles to the reflection pool at the bottom of Amicalola Falls. The Mountain Laurel Trail connects to the Base of Falls Trail and makes a loop of its own. Other paths tread along Little Amicalola Creek, which is stocked with trout during the warm season. The Appalachian Trail Approach leaves the visitor center, passes the lodge, and heads 8 miles to Springer Mountain. Or take the trail to the park's Hike Inn, an overnight destination that you may want to try. A 5-mile hike leads to this rustic getaway, set on a ridge at 3,100 feet.

During an interview, the park manager strongly emphasized the nature programs at this state park. They average seven programs per day, plenty to keep you busy and learning. Go on a tree identification hike, learn about insects, pioneer crafts, wilderness survival, and fire building. Other events include hayrides, nature bingo, movie shows, hoedowns, and scavenger hunts. This is great fun for kids and adults. Don't leave here without enjoying at least one of these events!

If you're feeling lazy and don't want to cook, the park lodge has buffet-style breakfasts, lunches, and dinners. You can actually walk from the campground to the lodge to grab your meal, burning at least a few of the calories that you will consume. On second thought, you may want to drive, in case you get too full—knowing that there are other calorie-consuming activities all over the state park with the tallest waterfall in the East.

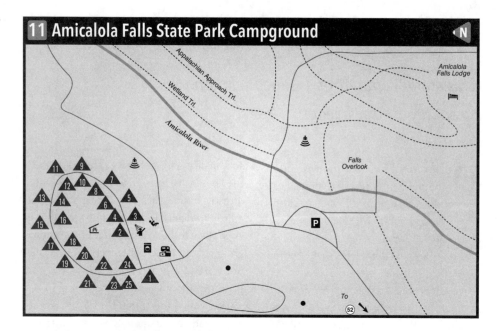

:: Getting There

From the town square in Dawsonville, take GA 53 West 3 miles to GA 183. Turn right on GA 183 and follow it 10 miles to GA 52. Turn right on GA 52 and follow it 1.5 miles to the state park, on your left.

GPS COORDINATES   N34° 34' 7.66"   W84° 14' 44.26"

12

Andrews Cove Campground

This small campground is located along a cool mountain stream.

During my numerous travels amid the mountains of northern Georgia, I can't tell you how many times I passed Andrews Cove Campground without stopping. It wasn't until I started systematically combing the state for this guidebook that Andrews Cove finally made my radar screen. And what an oversight I had made! This little campground packs a punch. Set in a richly wooded cove on Andrews Creek, flanked by Rocky Mountain to the north and Crumbly Knob to the south, "the little campground that could" provides a waterside getaway in the shadow of the Appalachian Trail, where trout fishing is the cast of a line away and the mountain town of Helen is accessible—but not too close.

Be prepared when approaching this campground on GA 75—the campground entrance is on a sharp, steep curve. What else would you expect in the mountains, though? The camping area begins shortly after leaving the paved road. The sky darkens overhead as a lush forest shadows Andrews Creek, a rocky and crystalline

:: Ratings

BEAUTY: ★ ★ ★ ★
PRIVACY: ★ ★ ★
SPACIOUSNESS: ★ ★ ★
QUIET: ★ ★ ★
SECURITY: ★ ★ ★
CLEANLINESS: ★ ★ ★

stream dropping amid rocks and boulders in the center of a cove. Site 1 is to your right, directly beside Andrews Creek. It may be a little too close to GA 75, but the camp is large. Reach the loop portion of the campground and turn right over a low water bridge. Site 2 is about as close as you can get to Andrews Creek without being in the water. Notice the tasteful rock and woodwork made to integrate these sites into the natural landscape. Trees actually grow out of the tent and picnic table pads, adding both shade and scenery. Native rock is left wherever possible without compromising a level camp. Site 3 is up the hillside and has a long "driveway." Actually, if you look closely, the campsite is set on an old roadbed. Pass the campground restroom. Site 4 is directly on Andrews Creek, which will sing campers to sleep at night.

Notice the tent pads—they are made of local stone and corral drainage-friendly pea gravel, yet another example of integrating the campground into the landscape. A spur road leads uphill to the next campsites. Site 5 is a little on the small side. Site 6 is backed into a hillside and is convenient for those wanting to hike the Andrews Creek Trail. Site 7 overlooks the lower camping area. Site 8 was my choice. I enjoyed its large size and its location backed against boulders on one side and Andrews Creek on the other.

The campground loop crosses back over Andrews Creek on a second low water

:: Key Information

ADDRESS: Chattooga Ranger District Office, 200 Highway 197 North, Clarksville, GA 30523

OPERATED BY: U.S. Forest Service

CONTACT: 706-754-6221, www.fs.usda.gov/conf

OPEN: Late March–October

SITES: 10

SITE AMENITIES: Picnic table, fire grate, lantern post, tent pad

ASSIGNMENT: First come, first served

REGISTRATION: Self-registration on-site

FACILITIES: Pump well, restroom

PARKING: At campsites only

FEE: $12

ELEVATION: 2,050 feet

RESTRICTIONS
- **Pets:** On leash only
- **Fires:** In fire rings only
- **Alcohol:** At campsites only
- **Vehicles:** 2 vehicles per site
- **Other:** 14-day stay limit

bridge to reach the final two campsites. These sites are much larger than the first eight and could function as double sites for larger families. They are in a flat along Andrews Creek. Wooden steps reach from the sites to the water. They also have wooden benches to accompany the outlined campsite "fixtures."

Other than the one restroom, a pump well serves the campground. With only 10 sites and a first come, first served policy, it means taking your chances. But other good tent campgrounds, detailed in this book, are nearby, should these sites be full.

Immediate campsite recreation includes trout fishing in Andrews Creek. Some land downstream—and all the land upstream—of the campground is national forest land, so fishing is doable without trespassing. Your best bet may be to head upstream. That way you can use the Andrews

Cove Trail to return to the campground. Be advised that the path stays well above the creek most of its 1.8-mile journey to meet the Appalachian Trail at Indian Grave Gap and FR 283. Northbound hiking on the AT will take you into the Tray Mountain Wilderness. Southbounders will hit Unicoi Gap. GA 75 crosses the AT at Unicoi Gap and makes for another access point. Water lovers should also consider heading north on GA 75 for 5 miles from Andrews Cove to High Shoals Scenic Area. The specially designated locale features the High Shoals Trail. It leads 1 mile first to the Blue Hole, a super-deep pool below an observation deck, then reaches High Shoals Falls—a cascade in excess of 100 feet! This will provide stark contrast if you decide to visit the mountain town of Helen, about the same distance south on GA 75 from Andrews Cove, "the little campground that could."

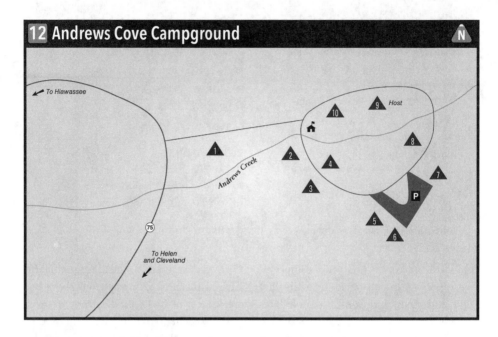

:: Getting There

From the bridge over the Chattahoochee River in Helen, take GA 75 North 6.5 miles to the campground, on your right.

GPS COORDINATES   N34° 46' 42.22"   W83° 44' 13.90"

13

Black Rock Mountain State Park Campground

Georgia's highest state park offers a tent-only camping section and plenty to see from atop Black Rock Mountain.

Black **Rock** Mountain Campground defies any campground stereotype—it has a 48-site campground with water, electricity, and cable TV hookups that is packed with RVs, but on a dead-end road on a mountaintop rib ridge is an 11-site, walk-in, tents-only area that complements the rest of the worthwhile sights and activities of the state park. The walk-in sites are the reasons this campground is in this book, and these are sites worth describing.

The walk-in sites are in three distinct areas. All sites are perched on the side of Black Rock Mountain wherever there is a hint of level ground. Some grading and site leveling have been done to make the sites camper-friendly. The mountain setting makes the sites incredibly appealing. Mix in some deep woods with far-off views, precipitous terrain, and a few cool breezes, and you have ridgetop tent camping at Black Rock Mountain State Park.

The main body of seven sites lies north of the parking area. Walk uphill and soon

you'll come to the first two sites, set off a bit from the trail for privacy. Thick woods separate all the sites from one another. The next five sites extend farther up the ridge, yet none are so far that you can't tote whatever you normally bring on a tent camping expedition. Just think of it as a little work to achieve the maximum in scenery and solitude. Sites D and E are downhill from the parking area, on either side of their own trail. Sites A and B have their own parking area and are even more isolated than the rest. Still, it's just a short walk back to the comfort station.

The comfort station stands beside the parking area. Inside, you'll find flush toilets, hot showers, and a dressing area for each gender. A water spigot is just outside the building. Ice, soft drinks, a washer and dryer, and a pay phone are back at the main campground. The Trading Post, which is the main campground store, has other supplies. That is the beauty of this setup: you can enjoy all these comforts but still camp in your own rustic atmosphere along with other tent campers.

Five mountains combine to make this the highest state park in Georgia. Black Rock gets its name from the sheer cliffs and outcrops of dark granite, called biotite-gneiss. For us that means open views of the Carolinas and Tennessee, as well as Georgia. Due to its high elevation, the mountaintop enjoys the same average summertime

:: Ratings

BEAUTY: ★ ★ ★
PRIVACY: ★ ★ ★ ★ ★
SPACIOUSNESS: ★ ★ ★ ★
QUIET: ★ ★ ★
SECURITY: ★ ★ ★ ★ ★
CLEANLINESS: ★ ★ ★

:: Key Information

ADDRESS: 3085 Black Mountain Parkway, Mountain City, GA 30562

OPERATED BY: Georgia State Parks

CONTACT: 706-746-2141, gastateparks.org

OPEN: Mid-March–November

SITES: 12 walk-in, tents only in season; 44 RV sites

SITE AMENITIES: Walk-in sites have tent pad, picnic table, fire ring; RV sites have water, electricity, and cable TV hookups.

ASSIGNMENT: May choose preferred site if available

REGISTRATION: Reservations required; call 800-864-7275 at least 2 days prior

to arrival; campers without reservations guaranteed one-night stay if site open

FACILITIES: Water, flush toilets, hot showers

PARKING: At parking area for walk-in sites

FEE: $20 walk-in, $30 RV

ELEVATION: 3,225 feet

RESTRICTIONS

■ **Pets:** On leash only
■ **Fires:** In fire rings only; must be attended at all times
■ **Alcohol:** Prohibited in public areas
■ **Vehicles:** None
■ **Other:** 2-day stay limit

temperatures as Burlington, Vermont. Interestingly enough, the Eastern Continental Divide splits the park. Water flowing off the north slope flows into the Mississippi and the Gulf of Mexico; the water from the south slope flows into the eastern seaboard of the Atlantic.

Speaking of water, there's a lake up there too. You can fish 17-acre Black Rock Lake from the bank for bass, bream, catfish, and trout. Boating and swimming are not allowed.

The most popular activity at Black Rock is hiking. Start out on the short Ada-Hi Falls Trail. The trail dips into a cool cove about 0.2 mile on the way to the falls. Because the trail and creek are so high on the mountain, there is not a whole lot of water to work with. Still, the trail will give you a taste of high-country woods.

Next, take on the 2.2-mile loop Tennessee Rock Trail. It swings through varied types of forest and tops out at the 3,640-foot peak of Black Rock Mountain. But the best view is a short way farther at Tennessee Rock. Look both ways at the countryside around you.

We came in late May; the high mountains around us offered varying tints of green as spring made its way up their crests. The valleys below were deep green. The shades became lighter with the rise in elevation. Tennessee Rock is a good place to catch a sunset. Another rewarding trek is the James E. Edmonds Trail, a 7.2-mile backcountry loop that traverses the north end of the park. A highlight of this trail is the view from Lookoff Mountain.

You'll find that Lookoff Mountain is only one of the many sights of this highland sanctuary in the North Georgia mountains.

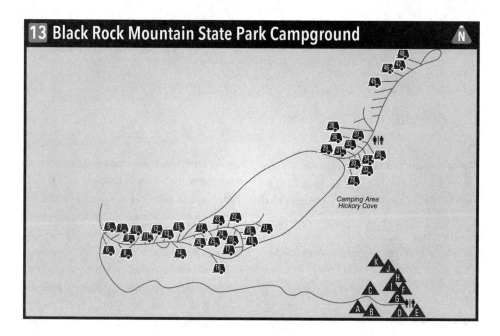

:: Getting There

From Mountain City take Black Rock Mountain Road west off US 441 3 miles. The road dead-ends at the park.

GPS COORDINATES   N34° 55' 2.78"   W83° 24' 39.75"

14

Cooper Creek Campground

Cooper Creek offers fishing, hiking, and camping in a designated scenic area.

They don't call it a scenic area for nothing—the Cooper Creek Scenic Area, that is. In this part of the Chattahoochee National Forest, a quintessential mountain stream flows beneath a richly wooded valley where white pines tower over rhododendron and hardwoods. Wildflowers bloom in spring and the high country air stays crisp in summer. Fall's colors contrast with the clear-green water frothing white over gray boulders and slowing in opaque pools, only to gather again and continue the inevitable course toward the sea.

Cooper Creek Campground is located on the edge of the scenic area, allowing easy access to the creek and its surrounding ridges. Favored by anglers, hikers, and those seeking to beat the summer heat and get back to nature, Cooper Creek delivers. Cross a bridge over Mulky Creek and enter the camping area. Site 1 is just beyond the bridge over Mulky Creek. It is on a hillside but has been leveled—as have all the sites—with landscaping timbers with gravel tent and picnic table pads. Site 2 is toward Coopers

Creek. Enter the main camping area, strung out on two half-loops centered by FR 236. Turn right to pass site 3, which is near the water spigot and is fairly large. Dip down to the coveted waterfront sites—4, 5, 6, and 8. Site 4 is worth the additional fee because it overlooks a pool in the stream. Site 5 enjoys the resonating sounds of Cooper Creek on a low bluff. A trail leads from here toward the center of the loop and restrooms. Site 6 also offers streamside camping. Site 7 is inside the loop. Site 8 is close to the stream but is partly screened from the water by laurel and rhododendron. Site 9 is away from the water but is unusual. It is a two-tiered site that accommodates a hillside. Site 10 is along an unnamed side stream feeding Cooper Creek.

The second half-loop leads away from Cooper Creek. Site 11 is on a hill all alone and is great for solitude. Site 12 has a long parking spur reaching another hilltop site. Sites 13–15 are the least desirable. They are on a spur road of their own but are a little too close to one another and a little too open. Sites 14 and 15 are so close as to function as a double campsite for small groups. Site 16 is large and level and is bordered by autumn olive bushes. Site 17 is reserved for the campground host in season. Water spigots are placed throughout the campground. Cooper Creek will fill starting the last weekend in March and then on nice weather summer weekends. Fall is a great time to visit.

:: Ratings

BEAUTY: ★ ★ ★ ★
PRIVACY: ★ ★ ★
SPACIOUSNESS: ★ ★ ★
QUIET: ★ ★ ★ ★
SECURITY: ★ ★ ★
CLEANLINESS: ★ ★ ★

:: Key Information

ADDRESS: Toccoa Ranger District Office, 6050 Appalachian Hwy., Blue Ridge, GA 30513

OPERATED BY: U.S. Forest Service

CONTACT: 706-632-3031, www.fs.usda.gov/conf

OPEN: Year-round; no water November–mid-March

SITES: 17

SITE AMENITIES: Picnic table, fire ring, tent pad, lantern post

ASSIGNMENT: First come, first served

REGISTRATION: Self-registration on-site

FACILITIES: Water spigot, vault toilets

PARKING: At campsites only

FEE: $8, waterfront sites $10; winter $4, waterfront sites $5

ELEVATION: 2,230 feet

RESTRICTIONS
- **Pets:** On leash only
- **Fires:** In fire rings only
- **Alcohol:** At campsites only
- **Vehicles:** 2 vehicles per site
- **Other:** 14-day stay limit

If you want to explore the Cooper Creek Scenic Area on foot, trails are just a few feet from the campground, near campsite 10. Here, the Millshoals Trail leads to a network of other paths. After 0.6 mile the Millshoals Trail meets the Cooper Creek Trail, a short connector path, then keeps going toward Millshoals Creek near FR 39. Curve around to meet Shope Gap Trail. Complete a loop on the Yellow Mountain Trail. A shorter loop is possible using the Cooper Creek Trail. The Yellow Mountain Trail also leads to Addie Gap. More possibilities can be seen on the hiking map at the trailhead.

You can head just a short distance down FR 236 to the Cooper Creek Scenic Area parking area and walk a fisherman's trail up Cooper Creek. Anglers will be banging through the laurel and rhododendron, going after brown and rainbow trout. Other anglers will head upstream from the campground and work their way to the scenic area parking area. Another interpretive trail, the Eyes on Wildlife Trail, leaves from this parking area. It makes a 1.3-mile loop, traversing many wildlife habitats, including a couple of wildlife openings, grassy plots in the forest designed to increase food for nature's beasts. The wildlife of Cooper Creek only serves to enhance the attractive scenery of this mountain stream, a designated scenic area.

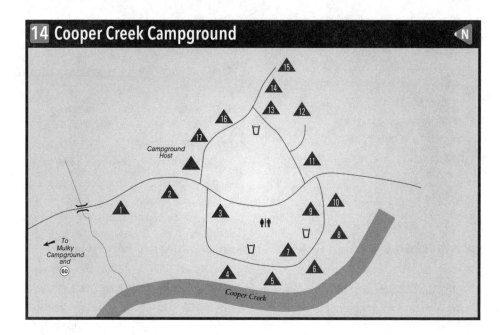

:: Getting There

From Blue Ridge, take US 76 East 4 miles to GA 60. Turn right on GA 60 and follow it south 18 miles to Cooper Creek Road. Turn left on Cooper Creek Road and follow it 5.2 miles to FR 236. Turn right on FR 636 and follow it 0.2 miles to the campground.

GPS COORDINATES   N34° 45' 46.45"   W84° 04' 4.63"

15

Deep Hole Campground

*The Toccoa River is the setting for this angler's
and canoer's campground.*

The Toccoa River is the primary draw at Deep Hole Campground. The campground takes its name from a hole of deep water in this stream that courses through Georgia's mountains. The alluring, greenish-clear water of the Toccoa crashes over rocks and boulders in shallow rapids but is broken by this slow-moving deep stretch beside the campground. Trout lurk in the depths and draw anglers eager to battle these cold water-loving fish. The Toccoa also draws paddlers, who like to tackle the class II rapids. Canoeing and kayaking are other ways to fish here. However, in my opinion, the river overshadows a beautiful campground that deserves some accolades of its own.

The campground is laid out in a loop—nothing special about that. It's the overall setting—an appealing forest highlighted by towering white pines spread over a streamside flat with maples, beech, and numerous dogwood trees as an understory, all near the Toccoa River. Adequate brush screens most campsites from each other. Boulders and wood posts delineate each camping area. Site 1 is the most open. It has younger hardwoods surrounding it. Site 2 is outside the loop. Hardwoods shade site 3. Site 4 is inside the loop and is shaded by pines and hardwoods. Site 5 is the most coveted and is the only streamside site. It is on a small bluff directly overlooking the Toccoa. Sites 6–8 are all inside the loop. Site 6 is large and deeply shaded by white pines. Site 7 is a little on the small side but has shade aplenty and is close to the fishing access (more about fishing later). I stayed in campsite 8. It was also near the fishing access and, truth be known, was also the only site available. It worked for me. Two sets of vault toilets serve the campground. This year-round campground fills on the opening weekend of trout season, the last weekend in March, and many nice weather weekends during the summer. However, if you arrive by midday Friday you should get a campsite, except for summer holiday weekends.

Fishing is the primary draw here at Deep Hole. The Georgia Department of Natural Resources (DNR) regularly stocks the Toccoa River. Near the campground, just above the Deep Hole, you will see a plastic tube leading into the water. This is where the trout are dropped down the tube and into the Toccoa. A fishing access has been built over the Deep Hole. From a concrete deck, anglers can toss a line over the rail into the water. Others will be wearing waders in spring, fishing directly in the river for rainbow trout. A canoe access is

:: Ratings

BEAUTY: ★ ★ ★ ★
PRIVACY: ★ ★ ★
SPACIOUSNESS: ★ ★ ★ ★
QUIET: ★ ★ ★ ★
SECURITY: ★ ★ ★
CLEANLINESS: ★ ★ ★

:: Key Information

ADDRESS: Toccoa Ranger District Office, 6050 Appalachian Hwy., Blue Ridge, GA 30513	**REGISTRATION:** Self-registration on-site
	FACILITIES: Vault toilet
OPERATED BY: U.S. Forest Service	**PARKING:** At campsites only
CONTACT: 706-632-3031, www.fs.usda.gov/conf	**FEE:** $10, waterfront sites $12
	ELEVATION: 1,975 feet
OPEN: Year-round	
SITES: 8	**RESTRICTIONS**
SITE AMENITIES: Picnic table, fire ring, tent pad, lantern post	■ **Pets:** On leash only
	■ **Fires:** In fire rings only
	■ **Alcohol:** At campsites only
ASSIGNMENT: First come, first served	■ **Vehicles:** 2 vehicles per site
	■ **Other:** 14-day stay limit

located just below the Deep Hole, near camp-site 5. From here, paddlers can debark in the craft of their choosing and enjoy streamside solitude while heading downstream into class II rapids. The Rock Creek Road Bridge is 1.2 miles downstream. It is 5 miles down to the suspension bridge used by those walking the Benton MacKaye Trail. There is no auto access here, however. The next auto access is 3 miles farther to Butt Bridge. An all-day run will take you from Deep Hole to Sandy Bottoms in 14 miles, where the Forest Service has located a boat take-out. A map of the national forest comes in handy here. Bring your paddling skills and a fishing pole, for you will be angling less-traveled waters. The Toccoa is sometimes paddled from Cooper Creek down to Deep Hole, but the water is often too shallow. Many more river miles await below Sandy Bottoms all the way to Lake Blue Ridge.

If you are in the mood to hike, the Benton MacKaye Trail and the Appalachian Trail are within reasonable driving distance. You passed the Benton MacKaye Trail on the way in, at Skeenah Gap. I have hiked the entire Benton MacKaye Trail from Springer Mountain in Georgia to the Ocoee River in Tennessee and consider this path an admirable 90-mile alternative to the Appalachian Trail, especially for solitude lovers. The BMT extends north to Smoky Mountains National Park. Head south on the BMT from Skeenah Gap and traverse Toonowee Mountain, then loop back on FR 816. This loop is also good for mountain bikers. Head south on GA 60 to pick up the AT at Woody Gap. However, this is one campground where you may want to focus on water activities. Others may see the campground as I did, as a destination unto itself that deserves accolades of its own.

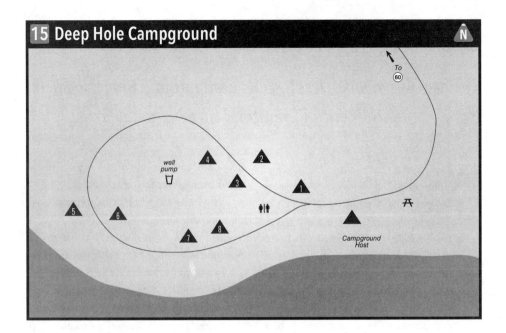

:: Getting There

From Blue Ridge, take US 76 East 4 miles to GA 60. Turn right on GA 60 and follow it south 17 miles to the campground, on your right.

GPS COORDINATES   N34° 45' 25.13"   W84° 09' 16.39"

16

Desoto Falls Campground

The heavily wooded Desoto Falls Campground is well located for exploring the central Chattahoochee National Forest.

Where do the names Desoto and Frogtown come together? The answer is at Desoto Falls Campground, which is located along the banks of Frogtown Creek in the 650-acre Desoto Falls Scenic Area. The sylvan campground provides a good base camp from which to enjoy the scenery of the falls, as well as the nearby Appalachian Trail and Raven Cliffs Wilderness.

With a campground this nice, it may be hard to tear yourself away. The 24 large campsites are split among two creekside loops arranged beneath a dense forest of deciduous and evergreen trees. It is one of the most densely forested campgrounds I've ever seen. This makes each site seem like an island unto itself and the campground seem more diffused than it really is.

The upper loop has a small stream running between the very spacious and private sites, which are separated by thick cover. Four low-volume flush toilets and two drinking faucets are interspersed in the loop. Seven sites border Frogtown Creek but are far enough back to be out of the flood-prone

areas. The intonations of the creek can be heard throughout the campground.

The lower loop has a campground host for campers' security. It also has several creekside sites. In the center of the loop is a modern restroom facility with warm showers. Two drinking fountains with connecting faucets complete this deluxe package. The campground has expanded its season and now extends from spring well into fall. Prices are lower during the shoulder seasons.

The primary attractions of this scenic area are the two falls located along Frogtown Creek. Why the name Desoto Falls? According to legend, early settlers found a strange piece of armor at the base of the falls. It was supposedly left behind by Hernando de Soto himself as he hunted for gold. Nearby Dahlonega actually did experience America's first gold rush in the 1830s.

The waterfalls of Frogtown Creek are natural treasures. The trail to the falls starts from the lower camping loop. Follow Frogtown Creek downstream 0.2 mile to view the Lower Falls drop some 35 feet onto the rocks below. Return upstream, past the campground, 0.7 mile to the Upper Falls with its four-stage, 90-foot drop. Be cautious as you tread the sometimes slippery trail.

Frogtown Creek and its tributaries offer quality trout fishing. Georgia Game and Fish stocks the stream weekly during the summer. Nearby Waters Creek offers special regulation trophy trout fishing.

:: Ratings

BEAUTY: ★ ★ ★ ★
PRIVACY: ★ ★ ★ ★ ★
SPACIOUSNESS: ★ ★ ★ ★ ★
QUIET: ★ ★ ★
SECURITY: ★ ★ ★ ★
CLEANLINESS: ★ ★ ★ ★

:: Key Information

ADDRESS: Brasstown Ranger District Office, 400 Wal-Mart Way Suite C, Dahlonega, GA 30523

OPERATED BY: U.S. Forest Service

CONTACT: 706-864-6173; **www.fs.usda.gov/conf**

OPEN: Year-round; no water or showers November–mid-March

SITES: 24

SITE AMENITIES: Tent pad, picnic table, fire ring, lantern post

ASSIGNMENT: First come, first served

REGISTRATION: Self-registration on-site

FACILITIES: Water, flush toilets, warm showers, drinking fountains

PARKING: At campsites only

FEE: $12, $6 winter

ELEVATION: 2,080 feet

RESTRICTIONS
- **Pets:** On leash only
- **Fires:** In fire rings only
- **Alcohol:** At campsites only
- **Vehicles:** 22-foot trailer length limit
- **Other:** 14-day stay limit

Just 1.5 miles up US 129 is Neels Gap and the Appalachian Trail. Either way you hike, you are in for a treat. We went both directions during our trip to the area. The wind blew hard during the 2.5-mile westward pull to the top of Blood Mountain. But the view from the highest point of the AT in Georgia was worth it. The rock outcrop of Blood Mountain, at 4,458 feet, enabled us to see far south into Georgia as clouds floated overhead.

We returned to Neels Gap for lunch, then headed east. First we passed Walasiyi, the state-owned hiking and gift shop. After perusing the unusual ridgetop store, we hiked into the Raven Cliffs Wilderness. The trail wound along the crest until we came to our destination at my favorite peak in Georgia, Cowrock Mountain. With a name like that, it had to be worth hiking 5 miles to see. And it was. The rock-overlaid peak offered views westward into the Boggs Creek watershed and summit after summit beyond that. We returned fulfilled to Neels Gap, then drove to Cleveland and devoured a well-deserved pizza that induced a sound night's rest back at the campground.

Towns Creek Trail (Forest Trail 131) and Dodds Creek Trail (FT 22) are two other pathways that lead into the heart of the 8,000-acre Raven Cliffs Wilderness. If you would like to know more about America's first gold rush, drive 4 miles south on US 129 to US 19, and then drive 12 miles to Dahlonega. The theme of this mountain town is the gold rush. They have some of the typical tourist traps, but also some worthwhile historic buildings and displays.

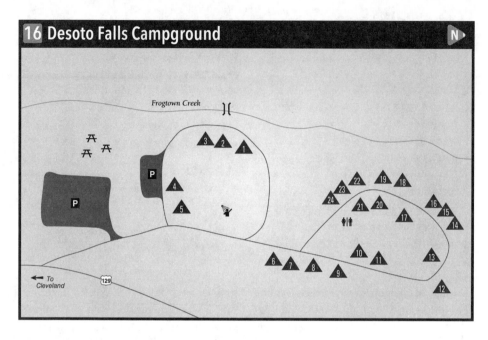

:: Getting There

Head north on US 129 from Cleveland 15 miles. Desoto Falls Recreation Area will be on your left.

GPS COORDINATES   N34° 42' 38.12"   W83° 54' 48.21"

17

Dockery Lake Campground

Relax in the highland campground beside the quiet waters of crystal-clear Dockery Lake.

An **exceptional** campground is set beside a trout-filled lake beneath the shadow of the Appalachian Trail. And that is only the beginning of Dockery Lake Campground. Tucked in a large cove on the southern shore of 3-acre Dockery Lake, this campground is as aesthetically pleasing as the natural mountain surroundings of the Cedar Ridge Mountain Range. The sites are landscaped using native stones with plenty of trees and ground cover that blend in well with the upland landscape. The tent pads are bordered in concrete with gravel pebbles for drainage. Not much leveling was needed, as the slope of the campground is negligible.

The sites are arranged on either side of a one-way gravel road, beneath a pine and hardwood forest with an evergreen understory. Five sites lie directly lakeside; the other six are only yards away but have the advantage of being high enough to overlook the lake. At the campground's end, a retaining wall encloses a small grassy area beside the lake, producing an ideal spot for fishing, sunbathing, or just relaxing.

:: Ratings

BEAUTY: ★ ★ ★ ★ ★
PRIVACY: ★ ★ ★ ★
SPACIOUSNESS: ★ ★ ★ ★
QUIET: ★ ★ ★ ★
SECURITY: ★ ★ ★
CLEANLINESS: ★ ★ ★ ★

Two combination water fountains and spigots are positioned around the campground, and a comfort station with flush toilets for each gender stands on the uphill side of the campground. The campground host resides at the campground's center, adding an element of security for visitors. The intimate lakeside environment spells vacation for any camper whose destination is Dockery Lake.

Dockery Lake is fed from the chilly headwaters of Waters Creek, tumbling off the slopes of Jacobs Knob along the Appalachian Trail. The pure water is sufficiently cold to support a healthy population of trout, so it comes as no surprise that fishing is a popular pastime at Dockery Lake. The lake is stocked on a regular basis by the Georgia Department of Natural Resources. Anglers can be found here using a rod and reel lakeside or in a canoe or other small craft. No motors are allowed, however. The 0.6-mile Lakeshore Trail snakes around the lake. Short side trails leading to platforms at the water's edge provide good fishing and lake views. A wooden platform with handrails sits over the small dam. It's a good vantage point for lake enthusiasts to take in the entire 6 acres of the crystalline body of water. The trail is graveled throughout the campground.

The one-way gravel road bisecting the campground leads a short distance to the picnic parking area. It is there that the Dockery Lake Trail begins. It leads 3.4 miles up to

:: Key Information

ADDRESS: Brasstown Ranger District Office, 400 Wal-Mart Way Suite C, Dahlonega, GA 30533

OPERATED BY: U.S. Forest Service

CONTACT: 706-864-6173; www.fs.usda.gov/conf

OPEN: Mid March–December; no water November and December

SITES: 11

SITE AMENITIES: Tent pad, fire ring, picnic table, lantern post

ASSIGNMENT: First come, first served

REGISTRATION: Self-registration on-site

FACILITIES: Water spigots, flush toilets

PARKING: At campsites

FEE: $8, $4 November and December

ELEVATION: 2,400 feet

RESTRICTIONS
- **Pets:** On leash only
- **Fires:** In fire rings only
- **Alcohol:** At campsites only
- **Vehicles:** 22-foot trailer length limit
- **Other:** 14-day stay limit

Miller Gap and the Appalachian Trail. Look for deer and grouse feeding in the shadows. After a mile of trail treading along tributaries of Waters Creek, you'll be lower than when you started. The trail climbs for the remainder of its journey to Miller Gap, just shy of 3,000 feet. It is 2.9 miles west on the AT to Woody Gap and GA 60. It is just over 5 miles east to Blood Mountain, at 4,458 feet, the highest point of the AT in Georgia.

For a scenic overview of the surrounding mountains, drive back to GA 60 and turn right. A quarter-mile on your right is the Chestatee Overlook, a cleared area offering a vista of the Chattahoochee National Forest to the east. Another mile up GA 60 is Woody Gap and a view of the Yahoola Valley. The AT passes through the grassy gap. If you need supplies, drive back to Dahlonega.

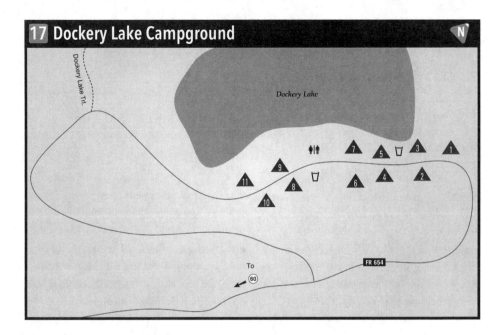

:: Getting There

From Dahlonega take GA 60 North 12 miles. Turn right at the sign for Dockery Lake on FR 654 for 1 mile.

GPS COORDINATES   N34° 40' 27.10"   W83° 58' 32.37"

18

Fort Yargo State Park Campground

The walk-in tent sites overlook Marbury Watershed Lake, the center of action here.

This state park follows the classic example of how many modern recreation areas have evolved. First, the future park area is the site of a historic event or structure. In this case, a small log fort was erected in the late 1700s as protection for early pioneers moving into the area. Over time, the structure goes through varying ownerships and stages of care before its historic relevance is realized. Then the area is preserved and the domain is given over or sold to a public entity. Finally, the public entity, in this case the state of Georgia, develops the historic site and adds recreation components for public use and, in this case, a fine campground on the shores of Marbury Watershed Lake was born.

The campground is broken into three parts—two drive-up camping loops and the walk-in tent-camping area. The first loop, Campground 1, contains sites 1–27. This recently renovated loop is situated in too-open pine woods and is the least desirable of the options. The sites have been nicely developed with gravel and landscaping timbers but were obviously built with RVs in mind. Several sites are waterfront, however, starting with 5–12. The remaining sites here are along a sloping hillside away from the lake. The sites there are larger and less popular than the lakefront sites.

Campground 2, with sites 29–40, is much better. The forest of pine, sweet gum, and oak is thicker, and campsite privacy is enhanced by more brush. The sites are widely dispersed and farther from the road. Dip down along a streambed where many sites are situated before passing a couple of waterfront sites. If you are going to use a standard campsite, go for these. Note that six yurts are located off this loop.

The waterfront walk-in tent sites are the best option. They are the most scenic and about half the price of the other sites. Leave the walk-in parking area and head out on a peninsula. Pines primarily shade the campsites. Rocks and large boulders are embedded into the forest floor. The campsites have been leveled around the rocky features and become more popular as you head out on the peninsula, which narrows to a point. Eight of the walk-in sites are waterfront. There is a comfort station with showers located in the walk-in tent area.

Other comfort stations with showers are conveniently located for all campers.

:: Ratings

BEAUTY: ★ ★ ★
PRIVACY: ★ ★ ★
SPACIOUSNESS: ★ ★ ★ ★
QUIET: ★ ★ ★ ★
SECURITY: ★ ★ ★ ★ ★
CLEANLINESS: ★ ★ ★ ★

:: Key Information

ADDRESS: P.O. Box 764, Winder, GA 30680

OPERATED BY: Georgia State Parks

CONTACT: 770-867-3489, **gastateparks .org;** reservations 800-864-7275

OPEN: Year-round

SITES: 12 walk-in, 40 other

SITE AMENITIES: Walk-in sites have picnic table, fire ring, tent pad, lantern post; others also have water and electricity

ASSIGNMENT: First come, first served or by reservation

REGISTRATION: At park office

FACILITIES: Hot showers, flush toilets

PARKING: At walk-in tent parking and at campsites

FEE: $24 walk-in sites, $28–30 all others

ELEVATION: 850 feet

RESTRICTIONS
- **Pets:** On leash only
- **Fires:** In fire rings only
- **Alcohol:** At campsites only
- **Vehicles:** 2 vehicles per site
- **Other:** 14-day stay limit

Being located between Athens and Atlanta puts heavy camping pressure on this park. It fills nearly every weekend from spring through fall. Reservations are in order here.

Marbury Watershed Lake, 260 acres, is not only the primary feature of the campground but is the centerpiece of the park. Fishing, boating, and swimming are popular. Warm-water species, such as bass, crappie, and bluegill, are sought after. A 10-horsepower limit keeps bigger boats and personal watercraft off the water yet allows anglers to cast their lines along the surprisingly large amount of shoreline. A boat ramp is located near the campground, as are two fishing piers. The swim beach is just across the lake at Day Use Area A. This is also where johnboats, pedal boats, and canoes can be rented. Paths depart from here, including one that leads to an overlook near the beach.

There are two ways to visit the actual Fort Yargo—by car or by trail. The Fern Trail, open to hikers and bikers, leaves the campground, crosses the Marbury Watershed Lake dam, and swings around the south shore of the lake to reach the fort. The park nature center, part of Will-A-Way Recreation Area, was designed as an all-access area. Both handicapped and other visitors can enjoy this part of the lake, which also has a playground, miniature golf, game courts, and short trail. Anglers can be seen fishing from the bridge connecting the recreation area to the group campground. A separate road leads to a bank fishing area, adding more evidence that recreation is spread all along the shores of this lake.

The actual Fort Yargo, on yet another part of the lakeshore, offers insight into the past of Barrow County. It is amazing to look at this fort as a defensive shelter against the Creek and Cherokee Indians. This fort was in operation for less than 20 years and then was sold in 1810 and used by John Hill as a residence. His family cemetery is within the park confines. The Daughters of the American Revolution first took interest in preserving the site in the 1920s, and eventually 1,800 acres were purchased around the site. Marbury Creek was dammed, and today we have a park more than worthy of inclusion in this book.

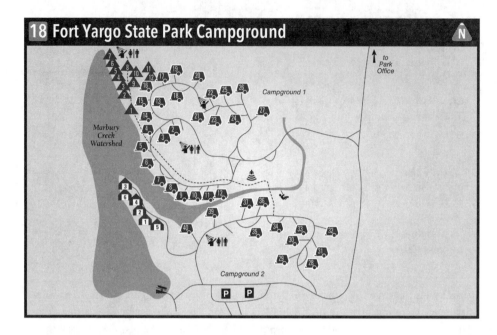

:: Getting There

From Barrow County Courthouse in downtown Winder, take GA 81 South 1 mile, then turn left into the campground.

GPS COORDINATES   N33° 58' 18.74"   W83° 43' 38.34"

19

Frank Gross Campground

This rustic camp is ideally located deep in the Chattahoochee National Forest, near trout fishing and hiking venues.

If you are looking to get way back in those gorgeous north Georgia mountains, here is your chance. Frank Gross Campground is in the back of beyond, along the upper stretches of Rock Creek, a mountain brook born high on the slopes of Greasy Mountain and Hawk Mountain, where the famed Appalachian Trail rolls out the first few miles after leaving its southern terminus at Springer Mountain. And Frank Gross is as primitive as the mountains—simple vault toilets, a hand pump well, and nature's primitive beauty all around you. Clear, rushing Rock Creek gathers in deep green pools where trout lurk, and steep forested hillsides rise from the flat upon which the camp sits. It seems surreal that the Chattahoochee Forest National Fish Hatchery is just down the gravel road, but it is, and ultimately that is a good thing, for it enhances Frank Gross. It does so by adding a place to see where trout are raised and also to check out some big ones. And a stream such as Rock Creek, with the hatchery being there, is going to be well stocked, which means more fishing fun for you and me!

On the way in, you will see dispersed camping areas. Angling campers are attracted to the fishing on Rock Creek, which travels beside Forest Road 69. Rock Creek becomes smaller above the fish hatchery, where Frank Gross is. Here, a simple gravel spur road enters a streamside flat. The campsite spur roads are also gravel. Site 1 is off to the right, close enough to Rock Creek that you can cast your line in from your tent. Site 2 is another coveted creekside site. They cost a little more but are worth it. A steep mountainside rises from the far side of Rock Creek, creating more "mountain effect." Site 3 is inside the loop, which is a combination of grass and trees. Site 4, like the others, is bordered with landscaping timbers to help keep it level. It is the most open campsite. Next is site 5, a streamside camp that has the added benefit of good shade. Site 6 is within steps of the pump well. Here, the campground road gets quite close to the stream and crosses a little brook feeding Rock Creek before reaching site 7, a streamside camp. Site 8 is the last camp beside Rock Creek and offers the best solitude. The last site, 9, is inside the loop and is the last campsite to fill. The vault toilets are on a hill across Forest Road 69. This place is first come, first served way back in the mountains, so you take a chance coming here. However, if it is full, you can go for a dispersed campsite along lower Rock Creek.

:: Ratings

BEAUTY: ★ ★ ★
PRIVACY: ★ ★ ★
SPACIOUSNESS: ★ ★ ★ ★
QUIET: ★ ★ ★ ★
SECURITY: ★ ★ ★
CLEANLINESS: ★ ★ ★

:: Key Information

ADDRESS: Toccoa District Ranger Station, 6050 Appalachian Hwy., Blue Ridge, GA 30513

OPERATED BY: U.S. Forest Service

CONTACT: 706-632-3031, www.fs.usda.gov/conf

OPEN: Late March–October

SITES: 9

SITE AMENITIES: Picnic table, fire ring, tent pad

ASSIGNMENT: First come, first served

REGISTRATION: Self-registration on-site

FACILITIES: Vault toilets

PARKING: At campsites only

FEE: $8

ELEVATION: 2,300 feet

RESTRICTIONS
- **Pets:** On leash only
- **Fires:** In fire rings only
- **Alcohol:** At campsites only
- **Vehicles:** 2 vehicles per site
- **Other:** 14-day stay limit

Fishing is a natural venue here. Just below the campground, a small dam backs up Rock Creek and avails a chance to fish a deep hole or even take a dip in cool Rock Creek if nobody is fishing there. Just downstream from the dam, at the upper end of the hatchery, Mill Creek enters Rock Creek. A spur trail goes up Mill Creek and offers backcountry trout fishing for stocked and wild trout for those who want to angle a tight canopied mountain stream, in an experience as primitive as Frank Gross Campground. You may want to tour the hatchery to get your angler juices flowing. It is open Monday–Friday, 7:30 a.m.–3:30 p.m. Annually, the hatchery distributes 324,000 catchable trout and also releases more than 400,000 fingerlings. That's a lot of fish! And many of them go in Rock Creek.

If you want to hike a little bit, simply drive up Forest Road 69 beyond Frank Gross to reach Hightower Gap, elevation 2,847 feet, and the crest of the mountains. Here, the famed Appalachian Trail crosses FR 69. It is 8 miles southbound to reach Springer Mountain and the end of the trail. A more realistic hike is to head southbound over Hawk Mountain, with a side trip to the Hawk Mountain trail shelter, then continue on to Forest Road 251, for an out-and-back trip of 4.6 miles. A good northbound hike would be to head toward Sassafras Mountain, reaching an overlook after 2.5 miles, for a round trip of 5 miles. Either way, a taste of the Appalachian Trail is likely to enhance your experience at Frank Gross Campground.

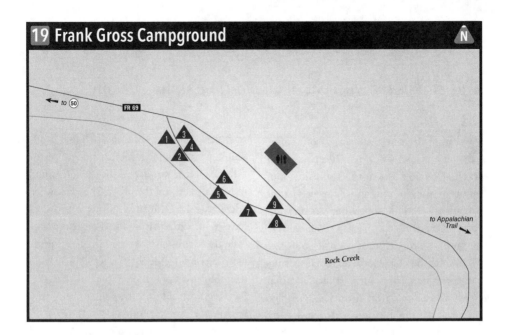

:: Getting There

From Dahlonega, take GA 60 north 28 miles to reach Rock Creek Road and the signed left turn for the Chattahoochee Forest National Fish Hatchery. Turn left on paved Rock Creek Road and follow it as it turns gravel after 1 mile. Continue forward as the gravel road becomes Forest Road 69. Follow FR 69 4 more miles, passing the fish hatchery. Frank Gross Campground is 0.2 mile beyond the hatchery on your right.

GPS COORDINATES   N34° 41' 58.57"   W84° 08' 44.44"

20

Hart State Park Campground

This park is reminiscent of an old-time summer camp.

This state park is a waterfront camping and recreation park destination of the first order. Most of the campsites (and all of the walk-in tent sites) are waterfront, and nearly all the fun here centers on water recreation. For that matter, you couldn't get away from the water even if you tried. The water here is Hartwell Lake, a huge impoundment damming the Savannah River. The Savannah is formed at this lake primarily by the Tugaloo and Keowee Rivers. Though most of the lake is in South Carolina, Georgia claims enough shoreline to establish this state park, naturally named Hart, in this area where it seems everything is named Hart, including the nearby town of Hartwell and the county in which this park lies, Hart County.

The campground has a wide variety of campsites, many of which are suitable for tent campers. The camping area as a whole is set on a hilly peninsula of Lake Hartwell. The first area, with sites 1–9, is near the water and for RVs. Sites 10–37 are mostly strung along the shoreline. Most of these sites are average in size and shade is limited, especially on the sites that have been

:: Ratings

BEAUTY: ★ ★ ★
PRIVACY: ★ ★
SPACIOUSNESS: ★ ★ ★
QUIET: ★ ★ ★
SECURITY: ★ ★ ★ ★ ★
CLEANLINESS: ★ ★ ★ ★

reworked. This reworking includes landscaping timbers for leveling and site restoration, a lower wooden platform with wood railings directly on the water. The woodwork adds appeal to the sites. Some of the sites have a dock exclusively for their use. However, these sites are too close together for my taste and are decidedly RV HQ. The ones on the point overlook a busy part of the lake. Starting with site 30, the sites overlook a narrow cove and are quieter.

The next loop is on a hill above the lower loop. It has sites 38–54, plus four primitive sites. The sites are in thicker yet younger woods of hickory, oak, dogwood, and pine. More brush adds privacy. These sites are more suitable for a tent, and the pads have been leveled. The primitive sites have no water and electricity and are good tent sites. The bathhouse is up on this loop.

The best in tent camping at Hart State Park are the waterfront tent-camping sites, sites 61–76 (sites 56–60 have sewer connections and are pure RV and therefore not desirable). These 16 tent sites are all waterfront and have water and electricity. The walk from your car to the sites does not exceed 30 yards. Most are decently shaded, though a few have limited shade. All sites are directly on the water. Understory is nonexistent.

The longest peninsula at this state park is reserved for recreation, including a large picnic area, swim beach, and open lawns. Basketball and volleyball courts and a horseshoe pit keep inland campers busy. The park

:: Key Information

ADDRESS: 330 Hart State Park Rd., Hartwell, GA 30643

OPERATED BY: Georgia State Parks

CONTACT: 706-376-8756, **gastateparks.org**

OPEN: March–September

SITES: 16 walk-in tent, 9 drive-up tent, 4 primitive, 47 RV sites

SITE AMENITIES: Picnic table, fire ring, lantern post, tent pad, water, electricity

ASSIGNMENT: First come, first served

REGISTRATION: At campground office

FACILITIES: Hot showers, flush toilets, laundry

PARKING: At walk-in tent-camper parking and campsites

FEE: $19 walk-in, $19–26 all others

ELEVATION: 660 feet

RESTRICTIONS

■ **Pets:** On leash only
■ **Fires:** In fire rings only
■ **Alcohol:** At campsites only
■ **Vehicles:** 2 vehicles per site
■ **Other:** 14-day stay limit

boat ramp is located here. Many, if not most, campers have boats.

During the warm season, this park can jump. The campground fills nearly every summer weekend, so get here early. Sites are available on spring, fall, and winter weekends and nearly every weekday of the warm season. At 138 acres, Hart State Park has a high density of users per acre. Beyond the borders, boaters will be on Hartwell Lake—skiing, tubing, fishing, and jet skiing. Bank fishing is fun and popular here. The park office sells bait and has fishing poles for loan. Inside the park, the boat ramps will

have boats loading and unloading. Kids will be splashing around the swim beach and plying the park roads on their bikes.

This park has the feel of an old-time summer camp. Campers, ranging from family groups to old friends and seniors, will be doing a wide range of things. If you are looking for a quiet getaway, don't come here. However, if you are looking for a fun-in-the-sun summer splash, then Hart State Park is for you. The town of Hartwell is nearby, food and supplies are readily available, and quick runs into town are part of the experience.

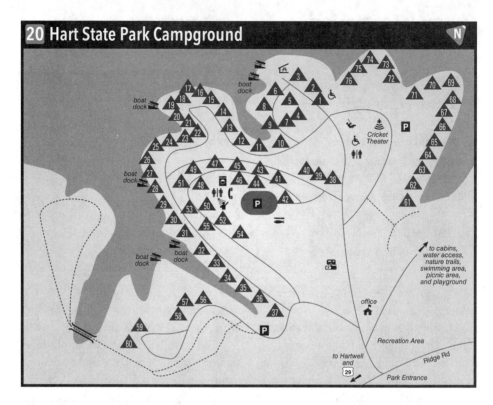

:: Getting There

From Hartwell, take US 29 North 1 mile to Ridge Road. Turn left on Ridge Road and follow it 1.4 miles to Hart State Park Road. Turn left on Hart State Park Road and follow it into the park.

GPS COORDINATES   N34° 22' 44.21"   W82° 54' 52.19"

21

Lake Russell Campground

This quiet, 100-acre lake is the centerpiece of a fine Forest Service recreation area.

Lake Russell is my kind of watery getaway. With 100 acres of water surface and a "no gas motors" policy, quiet is an integral component of the experience. With only 25 campsites spread over this long and narrow lake, the campground is never overcrowded. Hiking trails, great for walkers of all ages and abilities, emanate directly from the recreation area. Finally, Lake Russell not only has a picturesque swimming beach and good fishing but also a smaller impoundment, Nancytown Lake, which adds another watery element and angling destination to the Lake Russell experience.

The campground is divided into two loops that offer high-quality camping in distinctly different settings. Loop A, with sites 1–16, dips into a bowl-like hollow divided by a small stream. Tall pines shade the sites, alongside smaller trees, such as dogwood and sweetgum. The sites on the outside of the loop are cut into a hill but have been leveled using landscaping timbers. The sites inside the loop are large and set along the creek. Curve past the creek, and you'll find

more sites that are nicely separated. Tall tulip trees shade the loop here. This is one case where the sites inside the loop are best. Soon you'll reach the bathhouse and some of the most desirable sites. These sites, 12–14, require a short walk and are located closer to the lake. Site 16 is in a flat by the creek.

Loop B, with sites 17–42, is down the lake, on a ridgeline. The first sites are on a hillside away from the water. Some of the sites are integrated into the hill and are two-tiered. The sites are generally smaller but still plenty big for your tent and gear. The forest is thinner here but has adequate shade. The sites are well separated and located where the terrain permits, adding privacy. Curve toward the lake and come to some sites overlooking the lake and swim beach from hilly woods. Site 34 is of particular note, as it's the best in this area. Keep ascending the hillside to reach the end of the loop.

A campground host staffs Lake Russell. Three comfort stations and many water spigots are spread through the attractive campground. It will fill on summer holiday weekends and other nice weather weekends. Get here on Fridays by 2 or 3 p.m. and you should be able to get a site.

Lake Russell's alluring green water is stretched along a narrow valley encircled by pine-clad hills. Whether fishing or just paddling around, the scenery will leave you satisfied. The "no-gas-motors" rule keeps

:: Ratings

BEAUTY: ★ ★ ★ ★
PRIVACY: ★ ★ ★
SPACIOUSNESS: ★ ★ ★ ★ ★
QUIET: ★ ★ ★ ★
SECURITY: ★ ★ ★ ★
CLEANLINESS: ★ ★ ★ ★

:: Key Information

ADDRESS: Chattooga Ranger District Office, 200 Hwy. 197 N, Clarkesville, GA 30523	**FACILITIES:** Hot showers, flush toilets, water spigots
OPERATED BY: U.S. Forest Service	**PARKING:** At campsites and walk-in tent areas only
CONTACT: 706-754-6221, www.fs.usda.gov/conf	**FEE:** $12
OPEN: May–September	**ELEVATION:** 1,000 feet
SITES: 42	**RESTRICTIONS**
SITE AMENITIES: Picnic table, fire ring, lantern post, tent pad	■ **Pets:** On leash only ■ **Fires:** In fire rings only
ASSIGNMENT: First come, first served	■ **Alcohol:** At campsites ■ **Vehicles:** 2 vehicles per site
REGISTRATION: Self-registration on-site	■ **Other:** 14-day stay limit

your ears happy too. Anglers vie for bass, bream, and catfish on this lake. You passed Nancytown Lake on the way in. At only eight acres, this impoundment offers trout fishing in spring and a different watery setting. A carry-in boat launch is located here. Nancytown Lake is also the trailhead for some of the trails in the immediate area. The Sourwood Trail makes a 2.7-mile loop through rolling hills and past Nancytown Falls. The Ladyslipper Trail, open to hikers and mountain bikers, makes a 6.2-mile loop, traversing wooded hills and passing occasional vistas.

Lake Russell has one of the most attractive swim beaches in Georgia. Its well-manicured state reflects the entire recreation area. Picnic tables and a large changing facility stand atop a hill. Below, a lush grassy lawn leads to the equally appealing water. The Lake Russell Trail, which encircles the impoundment, can be used to access the swim beach and recreation area boat ramp from both camping loops. The 4.6-mile narrow path includes small bridges and attractive stonework and is a pleasure to walk. More than likely, your pleasure at Lake Russell will not be limited to the hiking trails.

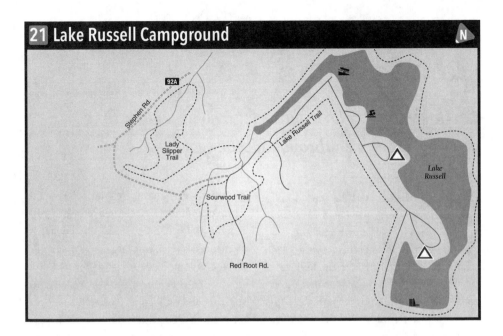

:: Getting There

Near Cornelia, take US 441 to US 411 Bus/GA 105 North to Wyly Street in Cornelia. Veer right onto Wyly Street, which turns into Dicks Hill Parkway (still a two-lane road), and stay with it 2 miles to Lake Russell Road. Turn right onto Lake Russell Road and follow it 3 miles to the campground.

GPS COORDINATES   N34° 29' 28.78"   W83° 29' 59.15"

22

Lake Winfield Scott Campground

This high-country lake makes for a good summertime getaway but is open throughout the year.

Lake Winfield Scott is one of those recreation areas that has a little bit of everything—a serene lake with fishing, boating for electric motors only, a swim beach, hiking trails that take you to the high country and the famed Appalachian Trail, and a good-quality campground, parts of which are open year-round. All of the above may be good, but what makes the overall picture better is the setting—the valley of Slaughter Creek, fed by small, clear streams coursing off the high ridges of Gaddis Mountain, Blood Mountain, and Slaughter Mountain. The campground and other facilities were tastefully integrated to maximize the area's natural beauty, resulting in a great destination for tent campers.

Enter the recreation area, reaching the South Loop first. The South Loop is open during the warm season. It is situated along Lance Branch, a feeder stream of Slaughter Creek. The sites here are very well separated by distance and are mostly screened from one another by ground vegetation. Pass the campground host site, then climb a hill, reaching sites 1 and 2. It is quite a distance to the next site on this large loop that could easily accommodate twice the sites. The only "loser sites" are 3 and 5, as they are too close together and on a slope. Sites 4, 6, and 7 are all desirable. Site 8 is a double site directly on Slaughter Creek and maybe worth paying twice the fee just for the solitude and setting. The loop curves along Lance Branch. Site 10 is all alone but near the bathhouse, one of two on this loop. Site 11 is near where Lance Branch and Slaughter Creek meet. Sites 13 and 15 are along the water and end the loop. Sites 16–19 are part of the group camp.

The North Loop, with sites 20–37, is situated along the valley of East Seabolt Creek. It is open year-round but has only a vault toilet and no water during the winter. The loop road is paved. The sites are large and well spaced from one another in a mix of pines, hardwoods, and evergreens. A healthy understory of mountain laurel, rhododendron, and younger trees screens the sites from one another. Reach a gravel spur road with sites 24–29. These are prime, shaded tent sites. Some are along East Seabolt Creek; others are cut into a hillside rising steeply away from the watercourse. All the sites have been leveled. I would pitch my tent here any day. Campsite 29 is at the end

:: Ratings

BEAUTY: ★ ★ ★ ★
PRIVACY: ★ ★ ★ ★
SPACIOUSNESS: ★ ★ ★
QUIET: ★ ★ ★ ★
SECURITY: ★ ★ ★ ★
CLEANLINESS: ★ ★ ★

:: Key Information

ADDRESS: Brasstown Ranger District Office, 400 Wal-Mart Way Suite C, Dahlonega, GA 30533

OPERATED BY: U.S. Forest Service

CONTACT: 706-864-6173; www.fs.usda.gov/conf

OPEN: North Loop open year-round, South Loop open late April–September

SITES: 37

SITE AMENITIES: Picnic table, fire grate, tent pad, lantern post

ASSIGNMENT: First come, first served

REGISTRATION: Self-registration on-site

FACILITIES: Hot showers, water spigots, flush toilets during warm season, vault toilet only in winter

PARKING: At campsites only

FEE: $15 North and South Loops, $7.50 North Loop in winter

ELEVATION: 2,900 feet

RESTRICTIONS
- **Pets:** On leash only
- **Fires:** In fire rings only
- **Alcohol:** At campsites only
- **Vehicles:** 2 vehicles per site
- **Other:** 14-day stay limit

of the road and is great for solitude lovers. An old roadbed continues beyond site 29 and is good for impromptu walking or wood gathering.

The main loop drops down along East Seabolt Creek. Large sites, some with pull-through auto parking, are open to the midday sun overhead. Site 30 is a double site close to the water. I stayed in site 32 during my wintry trip, enjoying the warmth of the sun during the early part of the day. A side trail leads to the lake and swim beach from site 37. The only drawback of this loop is that there's only one restroom serving it (near site 21).

Lake Winfield Scott draws most of the attention here. It has the amenities to go with the natural beauty of its 18 acres. A small dock allows easy entry and exit for small boats. The "no gas motors" rule keeps the atmosphere quiet. A fishing dock extends into the water near the lower end of the lake. Buoys border the wide and long swim beach. A rustic, large picnic shelter stands just in the woods by the swim beach.

The Lake Winfield Scott Trail extends around the lake and offers access for bank fishing or just to enjoy the vistas, especially looking across from the west side of the lake up at Slaughter Mountain.

In addition to the lake trail, other hiking trails leave from near the lake boat dock. An excellent loop can be made by heading up the Jarrard Gap Trail to the Appalachian Trail and the Blood Mountain Wilderness, then turning left, northbound, on the Appalachian Trail to Slaughter Gap, and back down Slaughter Creek Trail. A side trip to the top of Blood Mountain and its vistas is very well worth the additional effort. On my trip, the short winter day allowed only a hike up to Jarrard Gap, where I ran into some backpackers intent on making it all the way to Maine on the AT. The aforementioned and highly recommended day hike is 6.2 miles long, more than 2,000 miles shorter than the trip to Maine. After your day hike, you can return to your campsite in this recreation area that has a little bit of everything.

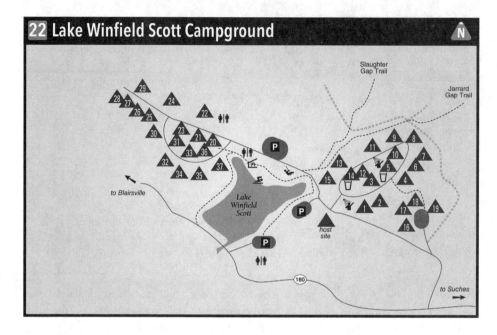

:: Getting There

From Dahlonega, take US 19 North 9 miles to Stone Pile Gap and GA 60. Veer left on GA 60 and follow it 7 miles to GA 180, Wolf Pen Gap Road. Turn right on GA 180 and follow it 4.4 miles to the recreation area, on your right.

GPS COORDINATES   N34° 44' 3.71"   W83° 58' 34.68"

23

Morganton Point Campground

This is your best tent camping option on beautiful Lake Blue Ridge.

Morganton Point Campground is located on the shores of Lake Blue Ridge, my favorite mountain lake of North Georgia. Maybe it's the memories, maybe it's the scenery. Maybe it's the alluring blue-green color of the water here. For whatever reason, it has earned a soft spot in my heart. I have had many adventures here, dating back to camping trips in a borrowed aluminum canoe, tenting on islands in the lake, looking out on high ridges rimming the horizon. The old canoe is long gone, but I still come back to Lake Blue Ridge. Walk-in tent sites located on a point overlooking the lake and other good sites combine to make an excellent base camp for exploring the lake and surrounding environs. Here, you can enjoy this high country lake, 1,700 feet, that takes a few degrees off the summer heat, and the nearby town of Blue Ridge, where the downtown has been revitalized with shops and such located on an historic street.

:: Ratings

BEAUTY: ★ ★ ★ ★
PRIVACY: ★ ★ ★
SPACIOUSNESS: ★ ★ ★
QUIET: ★ ★ ★
SECURITY: ★ ★ ★ ★
CLEANLINESS: ★ ★ ★

Morganton Point Campground is situated on a valuable spit of land facing south into Lake Blue Ridge. Pass the campground host, there for your safety and convenience, then move toward several nice drive-up sites, 1–7, in a hardwood forest, with most sites overlooking the lake. Enter the walk-in tent parking area. Beyond here, six shady campsites are set on a point that offers superlative views of Lake Blue Ridge. Sites A and D are a very short walk away, while the others require a mere stroll to reach the camps.

The campground continues in thick woods. The sites facing the lake are the most popular. Site 11 is of special note, as it is a lone walk-in tent site with a grand view. Go for this site first, if you can. The loop swings away from the lake and offers wooded, hilly sites that are attractive. The next area of the campground, with sites 20–37, is along a two-way road meandering through hollows. Some camps are wooded and isolated, such as sites 30 and 31, while others require steps and reach down to the lake, like 32 and 33. The rest of the sites are stretched along a dead-end road and offer great privacy but no lake views or access. This area is for solitude lovers.

A forest service boat ramp is conveniently located next to the campground. Anglers vie for bass, bream, catfish, and crappie on this 3,290-acre lake. Scenic boating

:: Key Information

ADDRESS: Toccoa District Ranger Station, 6050 Appalachian Hwy., Blue Ridge, GA 30513

OPERATED BY: U.S. Forest Service

CONTACT: 706-632-3031, **www.fs.usda .gov/conf;** reservations 877-444-6777, **recreation.gov**

OPEN: Mid-April–October

SITES: 7 walk-in tent sites, 37 drive-up sites

SITE AMENITIES: Picnic table, fire ring, lantern post

ASSIGNMENT: First come, first served and by reservation

REGISTRATION: Self-registration on-site or by phone or Internet

FACILITIES: Warm showers, water spigot

PARKING: At campsites and in walk-in tent camp parking area

FEE: $15

ELEVATION: 1,700 feet

RESTRICTIONS
- **Pets:** On leash only
- **Fires:** In fire rings only
- **Alcohol:** Prohibited
- **Vehicles:** 2 vehicles per site
- **Other:** 14-day stay limit

is also a pleasure, as most of the shoreline is owned by the forest service, lending it a natural aspect. A swim beach, located near the campground, is a big draw for campers and day users alike, though many campers swim along the shores in front of the campground. A trail leaves from the end of the campground, near campsite 37. The path cruises along the lakeshore. A picnic area overlooks Lake Blue Ridge. A boat ramp rounds out the recreation area facilities.

Other adventures require a little driving. If you are into hiking, the Benton Mac-Kaye Trail traverses the high ridges south of Lake Blue Ridge. To reach the BMT, take GA 60 south to the trail, which crosses GA 60. Take the BMT west from GA 60 and travel over Brawley Mountain, then back down to come near the Toccoa River after 3 miles. I have walked this ridgeline in complete solitude. From GA 60 going the other way, you have a crossing of Skeenah Creek, then a 1.9-mile climb to the top of Walallah Mountain. Call the Toccoa Ranger Station for a national forest map and more Benton MacKaye Trail information before heading out. A more civilized adventure will take you into the heart of downtown Blue Ridge. Get out of your car and walk around, browsing amid the shops located in restored buildings. A lot of good work has been done preserving this slice of Georgia's past. Hopefully, you will enjoy your adventure in this swath of North Georgia, making fond memories just as I have.

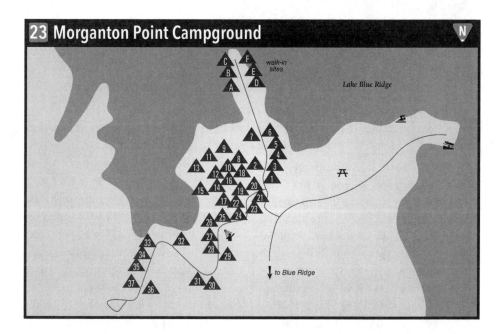

:: Getting There

From Blue Ridge, take US 76/GA2/GA 515 north 4 miles to GA 60. Turn right onto GA 60 south and follow it 1.8 miles to Bypass Road. Turn right on Bypass Road and follow it just a few feet, then turn right onto Lake Drive. Follow Lake Drive 1.3 miles to dead-end at the recreation area.

GPS COORDINATES   N34° 52' 6.68"   W84° 15' 14.45"

24

Rabun Beach Campground

This historic campground on Lake Rabun was built by the CCC in the 1930s.

Rabun Beach is a campground with a historic aspect. Back in the Great Depression of the 1930s, the Civilian Conservation Corps, a federal works program, was located here, building the infrastructure of not only this campground but also roads and other recreation areas of what was then part of the Nantahala National Forest. (Rabun Beach is now part of the Chattahoochee National Forest.) Today, you can enjoy not only an old-time campground but also Lake Rabun and the surrounding environment.

The campground has been altered a few times through its long existence, skewing the campsite numbering system. There are two major loops, each with a friendly campground host at the entrance. Area 1 has more vertical variation, as it is set along a small streamlet with hills rising from it. All the sites, 1–44, are nonelectric and offer both streamside and hillside environments. Enter the loop and you'll see a pretty and varied forest of white pine, dogwood, and maple, with lots of brushy mountain laurel and rhododendron. The first couple of sites are too close to Lake Rabun Road. Climb a hill into upland woods. These sites have been leveled and are a little more open and sunny. Come near site 15 and a connector road leads to Area 2. The main loop turns left and comes to more attractive sites, especially 21. Drop down to the streamlet, with sites 28A and 28C along the small streamlet. A dead-end road offers quiet sites 41–43 for folks who want to be on their own.

Area 2 has all of the electric sites. Enter the loop from Lake Rabun Road and enter a wide flat. This level locale was home to the old CCC camp. Spur B splits right and has sites 80–84. Most of these electric sites are too close to Lake Rabun Road. Of special note is site 80. It is notched all by itself beside a wet-weather stream and is nonelectric. Reach the loop with the bathhouse and sites 54–58 and 66–72. The loop is partly wooded with a mix of grassy and shaded sites. Finally, reach Spur A, with sites 60–65. These sites are higher, drier, and more piney. Water spigots and bathhouses are well spread throughout this loop. A connector road linking Area 1 with Area 2 has the Pear Tree Hill Group Camp and sites 49–53. The hillside sites have plenty of solitude. Campers at Area 1 must go to Area 2 for a shower. Rabun Beach Campground fills on summer holiday weekends. You should be able to get a campsite at other times.

Recreation is varied and immediately at hand. Lake Rabun is the big draw. This

:: Ratings

BEAUTY: ★ ★ ★
PRIVACY: ★ ★ ★
SPACIOUSNESS: ★ ★ ★
QUIET: ★ ★ ★ ★
SECURITY: ★ ★ ★
CLEANLINESS: ★ ★ ★

:: Key Information

ADDRESS: Tallulah Ranger District Office, 809 US 441, Clayton, GA 30525

OPERATED BY: U.S. Forest Service

CONTACT: 706-782-3320, www.fs.usda.gov/conf

OPEN: Late April–October

SITES: 60 nonelectric, 20 electric

SITE AMENITIES: Picnic table, fire grate, lantern post, tent pad

ASSIGNMENT: First come, first served

REGISTRATION: Self-registration on-site

FACILITIES: Hot showers, flush toilets, water spigots

PARKING: At campsites only

FEE: $14 nonelectric, $23 electric

ELEVATION: 1,950 feet

RESTRICTIONS
- **Pets:** On leash only
- **Fires:** In fire rings only
- **Alcohol:** At campsites only
- **Vehicles:** 2 vehicles per site
- **Other:** 14-day stay limit

reservoir is a dammed ribbon of water bordered by steep ridges curving through the Tallulah River valley. An appealing picnic area, shaded by white pines, is adjacent to the recreation area swim beach. A changing house overlooks the swim area, bordered by buoys. A floating dock is located within swimming distance of the shoreline. Benches are conveniently located so the elders can watch the younger set enjoy Lake Rabun. Boaters will be happy to know a launch is located just across Lake Rabun Road. Once on the lake, campers can fish for bass, bream, catfish, and trout. Boatless anglers do have a fishing option. The Forest Service has built a fishing pier on Lake Rabun. A short trail leads from the boat launch to the fishing pier.

The campground has its own hiking trail, the Rabun Beach Trail. It leads upstream along Joe Creek from near campsite 54. You will see a cascade just after crossing the first bridge, but this fall isn't even named. Reach the first named fall, Panther Falls, in less than a mile. Ahead is 65-foot Angel Falls. Joe Creek is a small stream and experiences low flows during late summer and fall, making the cascades a little less exciting, but the trail is a good leg stretcher, no matter how little water is flowing. On my visit, late spring rains left Joe Creek running high and noisy. The falls were the best aspect of an otherwise wet endeavor. All the same, I enjoyed my tent camping experience at Rabun Beach, as you will too.

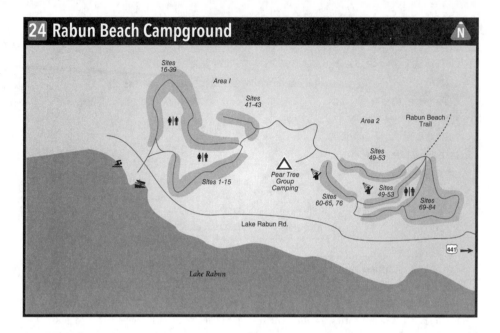

:: Getting There

From just north of Tallulah Falls, keep north on US 441 to Old US 441. Turn left on Old US 441 and follow it 2.5 miles to Lake Rabun Road. Turn left on Lake Rabun Road and follow it 5 miles to the campground, on your right.

GPS COORDINATES   N34° 45' 22.03"   W83° 28' 52.52"

25

Sarah's Creek Campground

This very primitive camp is set deep in the hills of Rabun County amid recreation opportunities.

Tucked away in a wide spot along Sarah's Creek, this campground occupies what was once known as Apple Valley. Sarah's Creek Campground "just kind of evolved," as it was explained to me. Locals had been camping here for years. Eventually, the Forest Service decided to develop an official campground. The improvement process continues. And if you place a high priority on getting back to nature on nature's terms, Sarah's Creek is just the place for you. It is located in an isolated area of the Chattahoochee National Forest in the extreme northeastern corner of Georgia, near the famed Chattooga River, the Bartram Trail, and Rabun Bald, at 4,696 feet the highest foot-only accessible mountain in the Peach State.

You don't have to worry about RVs coming to this campground. There are two ways to get in here, and each way is on a narrow road. Then out of nowhere, seemingly in the middle of nowhere, appears a grassy plot of land interspersed with shade trees and picnic tables! Primarily used as a hunting camp in fall, this campground is very lightly used

:: Ratings

BEAUTY: ★ ★ ★
PRIVACY: ★ ★ ★ ★
SPACIOUSNESS: ★ ★ ★ ★ ★
QUIET: ★ ★ ★ ★
SECURITY: ★ ★
CLEANLINESS: ★ ★

the rest of the year. And only a handful of the 25 sites appear to receive significant use.

Sarah's Creek exudes remoteness— there are no campground hosts. Some sites don't even have a picnic table and grill; some just have a fire ring with the table. You'll find no tent pads either. Just pitch your tent right on the flattest spot at your site. This is the most primitive campground in this guidebook. Not to say this place is ragged and neglected; it's just a work in progress.

When the Forest Service took over Apple Valley, they managed this part of Sarah's Creek for wildlife, planting autumn olive bushes and leaving a few clearings that still exist. The first five campsites border a clearing and are backed against wooded Sarah's Creek. Make a shallow ford and pass through a fast-disappearing clearing. Ahead, FR 155 leaves to the left. More sites are stretched beside FR 156, which continues along Sarah's Creek. A group of sites splits right on another ford. The clearing here has a campsite. Farther back are more wooded sites that border a tumbling feeder stream. The final two sites are located up FR 155 and offer great solitude.

Fishing is the only immediate recreation. The state stocks Sarah's Creek with trout during the warm season. However, Sarah's Creek makes a great base camp for the area's wilderness hiking, trout and smallmouth bass fishing, and forest drives. But a Forest Service map of the Chattahoochee is

:: Key Information

ADDRESS: Tallulah Ranger District, 809 US 441, Clayton, GA 30525

OPERATED BY: U.S. Forest Service

CONTACT: 706-782-3320, www.fs.usda.gov/conf

OPEN: Year-round

SITES: 25

SITE AMENITIES: Most have picnic tables, fire rings; some also have lantern posts

ASSIGNMENT: First come, first served

REGISTRATION: Self-registration on-site

FACILITIES: Vault toilet (bring your own water)

PARKING: At campsites only

FEE: $10

ELEVATION: 2,050 feet

RESTRICTIONS
- **Pets:** On leash only
- **Fires:** In fire rings only
- **Alcohol:** At campsites only
- **Vehicles:** None
- **Other:** 14-day stay limit

mandatory for making your way around.

To the west, just a few miles up FR 155, is the Bartram Trail. Named after naturalist William Bartram, the Bartram Trail begins on GA 28, east of Sarah's Creek on the Chattooga River at the Georgia–South Carolina border. It then travels southwest along the Chattooga, then north to cross FR 156, and on to its northerly terminus on Cheoah Bald, 37 miles in Georgia and 60 miles more in North Carolina. I have hiked the entire Bartram and think it is a superior experience to the Georgia portion of the Appalachian Trail. When ordering a forest map, also ask for information on the Bartram Trail.

Your closest access to the Bartram Trail from Sarah's Creek is on FR 155. Take the BT north from FR 155, and the trail heads around the west side of Double Knob, with far-reaching views to the north and west. Below lies Ramey Field. Across Ramey Creek is the rock face of Flat Top, where the Bartram Trail soon leads. Reach a gap between

Wilson Knob and Flat Top. Climb to enjoy a view to the south, of mountains fading into the Piedmont. Ahead, look for a side trail leading left to a fantastic view from a rock face, 2 miles from FR 155. Here, the horizon stretches southward from east to west. This view is so impressive that it made the cover of my book *Long Trails of the Southeast*.

The Chattooga River is to the east of Sarah's Creek Campground, simply one of the best rivers anywhere. Here, you can hike along the Chattooga, a federally designated wild and scenic river. Or fish for trout and smallmouth bass in a setting so spectacular that even fishless days are rewarding. If you haven't rafted the Chattooga, here's your chance. Several outfitters are located by the river off US 76. This has been one of my favorite rivers for a long time, whether it be for backpacking, fishing, tent camping, or rafting, and it is just one of the many recreation opportunities available here in Rabun County.

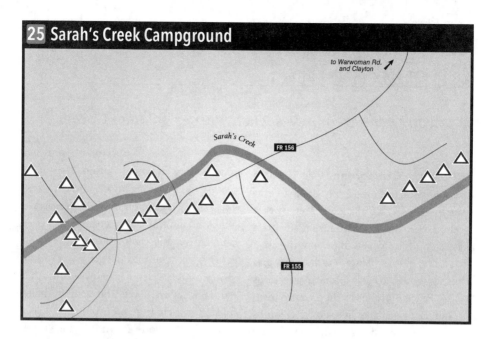

25 Sarah's Creek Campground

to Warwoman Rd. and Clayton

Sarah's Creek

FR 156

FR 155

:: Getting There

From just north of the junction of US 76 and US 441 in Clayton, head east on Warwoman Road and follow it 9 miles to Sarah's Creek Road. Sarah's Creek Road is on a downhill right curve and is easily missed. Turn left onto Sarah's Creek Road, FR 156, and follow it 2 miles to the campground.

GPS COORDINATES   N34° 55' 46.35"   W83° 15' 52.61"

26

Tallulah Gorge State Park Campground

You won't believe your eyes when you see Tallulah Gorge!

Terrora Campground at Tallulah Gorge State Park simply doesn't compare to the spectacular natural scenery that is the gorge. But it makes for an adequate base camp from which to explore the area. The Tallulah River Gorge, cut by water and time, is one of the most spectacular features in the Peach State. Near the historic town of Tallulah Falls, the Tallulah River drops deeply into a steep and scenic canyon, where waterfalls continue to cut the gorge ever deeper. And your exploration of the canyon begins with setting up camp at Terrora.

The well-maintained and staffed campground is laid out in a loop with crossroads. The sites are in good shape; however, unfortunately, they are close together. Plan on becoming friends with your neighbor. A younger forest primarily of oaks, dogwoods, and maples offer some shade. The auto pull-ins are gravel, but the camp road is paved. The campsites are graveled also. Two bathhouses serve the campground. You will see active campers here, with bicycles and hiking gear all poised to explore. There's not

much sitting around at Terrora. The campground fills on spring break, summer weekends, and gets close during fall leaf season.

A hiking trail leads to the interpretive center from the campground. Bring your camera with you into the gorge. Leave the visitor center, which has many historic and natural displays about the area. A helpful staff is there to answer you questions as well. Take the North Rim Trail where pines dominate the top of the gorge woodland. Soon reach Overlook #1. The overlooks are numbered to help you keep apprised where you are. The fallen tower beside Overlook #1 is the north tower used by Karl Wallenda to string wire across the gorge, which he walked across in 1970. The view is a long look into the deeper south end of the gorge.

Backtrack on the North Rim Trail, passing around the back of the Jane Hurt Yarn Interpretive Center. Descend to reach Overlook #3, and begin a loop on the Hurricane Falls Trail. Overlook #3 reveals LaDore Falls or L'Eau d'Or Falls, which is French for "water of gold." Begin descending the first of 750 steps to the suspension bridge over the Tallulah River, stopping at Overlook #2, which also has views of LaDore Falls. Admire the natural features that make the gorge so spectacular—steep-sided rock walls, sheer cliffs, crashing water below. Reach the suspension bridge and linger if you dare. Below you, Hurricane Falls makes its way over striated rock.

:: Ratings

BEAUTY: ★ ★
PRIVACY: ★ ★
SPACIOUSNESS: ★ ★
QUIET: ★ ★ ★
SECURITY: ★ ★ ★ ★ ★
CLEANLINESS: ★ ★ ★ ★ ★

:: Key Information

ADDRESS: P.O. Box 12, Tallulah Falls, GA 30573

OPERATED BY: Georgia Power

CONTACT: 706-754-7970, **gastateparks .org;** reservations 706-754-7979

OPEN: March–November

SITES: 50

SITE AMENITIES: Picnic table, fire ring, upright grill, lantern post, water, electricity

ASSIGNMENT: First come, first served and by reservation

REGISTRATION: At campground entrance station

FACILITIES: Hot showers, flush toilets, laundry, pay phone

PARKING: At campsites

FEE: $18 tent, $20 RV

ELEVATION: 1,700 feet

RESTRICTIONS
- **Pets:** On a leash
- **Fires:** In fire rings only
- **Alcohol:** Prohibited in public-use areas
- **Vehicles:** 2 vehicles per site
- **Other:** 14-day stay limit

Another set of steps wait across the river. Here, you get to take the 450 steps down to the bottom of the gorge. A viewing platform allows a bottom-up look at Hurricane Falls. To continue down the gorge, you need a permit, which can be gotten at the interpretive center. Only a finite number of permits are issued for descending the gorge. It is here, for those with permits, that the river can be crossed over rocks, if the river levels allow.

More climbing awaits as you make your way up to the top of the south rim. Tallulah Gorge has been a tourist attraction for quite some time, well before the state park was established in 1992, as a cooperative effort between Georgia Power and the state of Georgia. Reach the crest of the gorge and make your way toward Overlooks #8, #9, and #10. Look downstream for the interpretive center and across the gorge for a side stream waterfall, Caledonia Cascade, plunging into the gorge. See Oceana Falls from Overlook #9. Overlook #10 opens to Caledonia Cascade and a 1,000-foot bluff across the gorge. Overlook #7 looks over Tempesta Falls. Overlook #6 looks down the gorge. Overlook #5 opens to the upper gorge. Overlook #4 opens to the Tallulah Falls Dam, which was finished in 1913. From here, the trail crosses a small creek and soon comes to Overlook #3. Another good hiking venue is just a few miles south of the Tallulah Gorge, at Panther Creek, off US 441. It heads down a mountain canyon to end at Panther Creek Falls, another "gorge-ous" destination here in the swath of northeast Georgia. The park has other activities, too, such as swimming. A beach is open on Tallulah Falls Lake from Memorial Day to Labor Day. You can also paddle a canoe or kayak on the lake. The park has tennis courts, more hiking trails, and fishing. There, is so much to do here, you won't be spending much time at your campsite anyway.

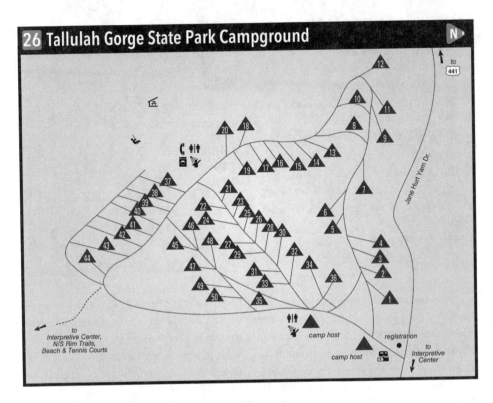

26 Tallulah Gorge State Park Campground

:: Getting There

From Cornelia, take US 441 north 22 miles to span the Tallulah River. Tallulah Falls Lake will be on the left on the bridge crossing. Shortly past the river and lake, turn right to enter the state park and follow Jane Hurt Yarn Road to the Jane Hurt Yarn Interpretive Center and Terrora Campground, which will be on the right after you enter the state park.

GPS COORDINATES   N34° 44' 29.34"   W83° 23' 46.12"

27

Tate Branch Campground

Enjoy streamside camping and wilderness hiking deep in the Georgia mountains.

Tate Branch, a small, streamside campground, lies nestled far back in the mountains of northeast Georgia. Tate Branch flows through the campground into the unspoiled Tallulah River, which provides a panoramic backdrop for your time here. Near the appealing campground are fishing opportunities, the Coleman River Scenic Area, and the Southern Nantahala Wilderness.

Tate Branch spreads all but five of its sites on a densely forested loop. Thickets of rhododendron produce secluded campsites. A campground host occupies the first site in the loop, next to the pay station, during the warm season. Seven sites lie by the Tallulah River, running about 30 feet wide at this juncture. The next five sites are between the loop and FR 70, which can be a little noisy from the sporadic traffic. Two very shady sites sit inside the loop, along with a vault toilet and an old-fashioned water pump. One site is located right off of FR 70.

What makes this campground different are the sites in a pine forest across from

FR 70. Just beyond a small parking area are four tent-only campsites. Though not that far from the primary campground, the four sites put like-minded tent campers together. Two of the sites lie fairly close to the road, thus requiring very little walking. However, the other two sites sit a little farther back and provide added seclusion. A small meadow lies between Tate Branch and the farthest site.

I stayed at the farthest tent-only site on a day that saw thunderstorms saturate the region. Light from the wildlife opening provided a cheery atmosphere. Yet I didn't stay in my tent and sulk. I donned my rain suit, grabbed a fishing pole, and headed back down FR 70 to the Coleman River Scenic Area. This 330-acre slice of the past is a remnant of the vast, old-growth forest that once cloaked the length and breadth of Southern Appalachia. I cast my lure into emerald pools below cascades that tumbled beneath giant boulders. I had no luck with the fish, but I wasn't paying that much attention as I walked along the Coleman River Trail; I was in awe of the white pines overhead. Drops of rain descended from branch to branch far above me, only to land on the ferns and rhododendron below. The trail dead-ended after a mile. So I turned around and took it all in from a different perspective.

The Tallulah River rose and turned murky after the storm. I drove along its lower reaches on the way to Clayton. I

:: Ratings

BEAUTY: ★ ★ ★ ★
PRIVACY: ★ ★ ★ ★
SPACIOUSNESS: ★ ★ ★ ★
QUIET: ★ ★ ★
SECURITY: ★ ★ ★ ★
CLEANLINESS: ★ ★ ★ ★

:: Key Information

ADDRESS: Tallulah Ranger District, 809 US 441, Clayton, GA 30525	**FACILITIES:** Hand-pumped water, vault toilet
OPERATED BY: U.S. Forest Service	**PARKING:** At campsites only
CONTACT: 706-782-3320, www.fs.usda.gov/conf	**FEE:** $14
OPEN: Late March–October	**ELEVATION:** 2,300 feet
SITES: 18	**RESTRICTIONS**
SITE AMENITIES: Tent pad, fire grate, lantern post, picnic table	■ **Pets:** On leash only ■ **Fires:** In fire grates only
ASSIGNMENT: First come, first served	■ **Alcohol:** At campsites only ■ **Vehicles:** 22-foot trailer length limit
REGISTRATION: Self-registration on-site	■ **Other:** 14-day stay limit

watched the river froth and boil between sizable boulders as fishermen hoped the "stockers" would take their bait offerings. Tallulah River is stocked with trout weekly during the summer. Back at camp, I mustered a fire from wet wood and warmed my bones as fog crept down the river valley.

The Southern Nantahala Wilderness makes for good exploration, also, because it is a rough, rugged, undeveloped area that straddles the North Carolina–Georgia border. This is a great place to hone your orientation skills by exploring old logging roads and unmaintained trails. However, two marked trails will provide a great hike from known position to known position—they also include great scenery. Get the Southern Nantahala Wilderness map at the Ranger Station in Clayton.

Continue up FR 70 until it crosses into North Carolina. FR 70 turns into FR 56 when it enters the Tar Heel State. Shortly after you cross the border, the Beech Creek Trail (378) begins on your right. The trail follows Beech Creek through the wilderness to the high country, passing an impressive unnamed falls as it veers toward Case Knife Gap and its high point. Then the trail switchbacks down to FR 56 and the headwaters of the Tallulah River. Take a short road walk back to your vehicle.

At the end of FR 56 is the Deep Gap Branch Trail (377). It leads 2 miles up the Appalachian Trail at Deep Gap. Just after you enter the wilderness, a short trail leads up a side branch at a falls. Check it out and return to 377. Head east on the AT and come to the Standing Indian shelter at 0.8 miles. Just 2 miles farther is the top of Standing Indian Mountain. To the east are the headwaters of the Nantahala River and to the west are the headwaters of the Tallulah River. From 5,499 feet, you can look into the Tallulah River gorge. Somewhere down there is Tate Branch Campground. After this hike, you'll be glad to call it home.

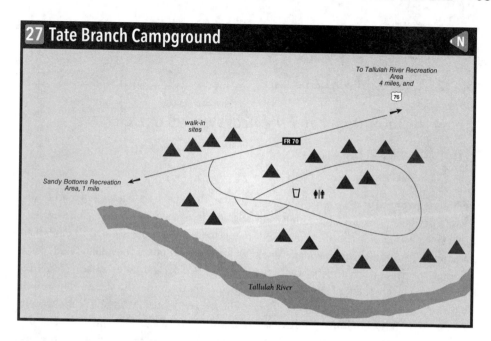

:: Getting There

Take US 76 West from Clayton 8 miles. Turn right on Persimmon Road and follow it 4 miles. Turn left on FR 70 4 miles. Tate Branch Campground will be on your left.

GPS COORDINATES   N34° 57' 24.62"   W83° 33' 9.91"

28

Unicoi State Park Campground

Enjoy the mountains and the nearby town of Helen from this state park.

Close proximity to a town might seem a detriment for a campground, but Unicoi State Park pulls it off. The mountain setting is immediately evident upon entering the park, which dispenses with the tourist-town atmosphere of nearby Helen. And easy access to town can be a good thing. You can enjoy the gastronomic smorgasbord Helen offers, from pulled taffy to cheese logs to foot-long hot dogs and more, and all the tourist offerings not involving food. The state park even has a hiking trail connecting it to Helen! That way, you can work off that food you ate in town. However, you may just want to explore the park, which has more natural attractions.

The campground offers many different options facility-wise, from the desired walk-in tent sites to the wooden platforms of the Squirrel's Nest, which you have to see to believe. First, reach Little Brook, with sites 1–16. White pine, hardwoods, and not much understory shade these water and electric

sites. The sites have been leveled and integrated into the hollow, but they are a bit close together. The loop dips sharply and then climbs steeply out of the hollow. Next, come to Big Brook, with sites 17–29. These full hook-up sites are along a stream and are well shaded but decidedly the land of the RV. Dip down, then come to tent-land, a.k.a. Hickory Hollow, with sites 53–85. These are laid out all over a hillside. Shade is adequate, and the sites are small to average in size. Understory vegetation is lacking. The first set of sites, 53–63, is preferable. These sites are more spread apart than the other section and are closer to the comfort station. Sites in the second portion, 64–85, are closer together and less wooded. Overall, these will do. Laurel Ridge, with sites 30–52, is next. These sites are too close together on a small ridge and are the least preferable of the whole campground.

The final camping option is the Squirrel's Nest. Park near the Trading Post and walk to reach a small hollow. A set of 16 platforms built together on the far hill look like the project of a young architectural student. But upon closer inspection, the platforms, each with roof, floor, and back wall, are interesting and the cheapest camping option. You cannot pitch a tent here, however. Just bring your camping equipment, and the wood roof will keep you dry! Water and a comfort station are nearby, as they are throughout the camping

:: Ratings

BEAUTY: ★ ★ ★
PRIVACY: ★ ★ ★
SPACIOUSNESS: ★ ★
QUIET: ★ ★ ★
SECURITY: ★ ★ ★ ★ ★
CLEANLINESS: ★ ★ ★ ★

:: Key Information

ADDRESS: 1788 GA 356, Helen, GA 30545

OPERATED BY: Georgia State Parks

CONTACT: 706-878-4726, **gastateparks .org;** reservations 800-573-9659

OPEN: Year-round; Little Brook and Squirrel's Nest closed in winter

SITES: 33 walk-in, 38 water and electricity, 13 full hookups, 16 wooden platform sites (Squirrel's Nests)

SITE AMENITIES: Picnic tables, fire rings, lantern posts, tent pads

ASSIGNMENT: First come, first served or by reservation

REGISTRATION: At camper check-in at campground in warm season, at lodge in winter

FACILITIES: Hot showers, flush toilets, laundry, trading post

PARKING: At walk-in tent site parking, Squirrel's Nest parking and at campsites

FEE: $25 walk-in, $29 water and electric, $35 full hookups, $15 Squirrel's Nest; rates may be higher on holiday weekends

ELEVATION: 1,700 feet

RESTRICTIONS
- **Pets:** On leash only
- **Fires:** In fire rings
- **Alcohol:** At sites
- **Vehicles:** 2 vehicles per site
- **Other:** 14-day stay limit

area. I plan on staying in one of these Squirrel's Nests when I return to Unicoi.

This is a busy park and fills often from spring through fall. Reservations are recommended. Camping here is a lot cheaper than getting a hotel in town or staying in the park lodge.

As previously mentioned, a path—the Unicoi/Helen Trail—will take you on a 3-mile walk through the woods to Helen. Mountain bikers can tackle a 7-mile loop designated just for them. This path also skirts Helen. The Lake Trail circles for 2.5 miles around Lake Unicoi. The Bottoms Loop explores the land around Smith Creek and is a good wildflower hike in spring. The Frog Pond Nature Trail has interpretive signs that help you learn about the park. There are two ways to check out nearby Anna Ruby Falls, on national forest land. You can take the Smith Creek Trail from the campground 4.8 miles one-way to the falls. If you drive, you can get within a half-mile of this cascade.

Swimming is a good way to cool off in the summertime. Campers have their own swim beach on Lake Unicoi. A separate swim beach for day users is across the lake. You can see the entire lake via a rented canoe or paddleboat and go fishing for catfish, bass, and bream. You can also fish Smith Creek for trout both below and above the lake. Check the latest regulations concerning trout fishing. Trout fishing is also popular in and around Helen on the Chattahoochee River. Tubing is also fun on this river. Outfitters are in town and rent tubes and provide shuttles for those who want to cool off in the 'Hooch.

This park prides itself on the interpretive programs they have. Take the time to join a ranger to learn about the flora and fauna of the northeast Georgia mountains. These programs include guided hikes, gold panning, and events just for kids. That way, you can balance your tourism time with a little nature time.

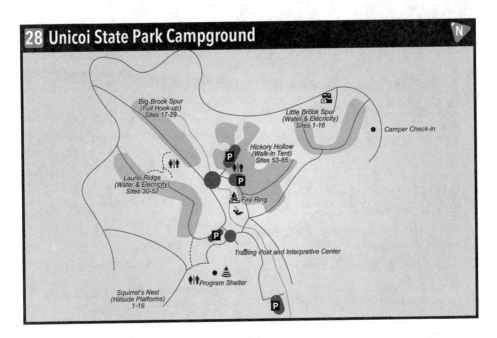

:: Getting There

From the Chattahoochee River in downtown Helen, head north on GA 75 1 mile to GA 356. Turn right on GA 356 and follow it 2 miles to the park. Turn left into the campground during summer to register. In winter, turn right into the lodge to register.

GPS COORDINATES   N34° 43' 28.48"   W83° 43' 37.85"

29

Upper Chattahoochee Campground

Camp beside the headwaters of Georgia's most famous river, the Chattahoochee.

Upper **Chattahoochee** is a favorite campground of mine in the Chattahoochee National Forest. And it seems the Forest Service has used all the positive things it has learned in the past to construct this campground. It is located in a long, level cove where the headwaters of the Chattahoochee River merge beneath the high ridges that form the northern border of the Chattahoochee River Basin. Georgia's most famous river flows beyond this campground southward through the state and on to the Gulf of Mexico. Here, deep in the mountains, the Forest Service has integrated the campground into the natural stage of wood, water, and wildlife openings, edged on three sides by the Mark Trail Wilderness.

The attractive campsites stretch out in linear fashion in three sections along a dead-end gravel road. The first group of sites sits in an open flat between the Chattahoochee River and Henson Creek. The second group's sites are dispersed on a short loop along Henson Creek. The third and largest section of sites is at the head of the cove. This arrangement produces a small campground feel, even though there are 34 units.

You can choose whatever woodland setting you please. Some sites are located in open grassy areas. Eight sites are nestled beneath shady trees and require a short walk. But no matter what site you choose, you are never far from the river or one of its feeder streams. Some sites even have stand-up grills, ready for charcoal and your favorite food. Simply put, there isn't a bad site in this campground, only a wide variety of sites. The five, rough miles of gravel road keep this campground from being overrun. During my stay in mid-May, I was the only person at the whole campground.

Three bathroom facilities with multiple low-volume flush toilets are adequately distributed. So are the three hand-pump water sources, which are combination water fountains and spigots. It's easy to recycle in the many recycling bins about the campground. For your safety, a campground host is usually stationed at the heart of the campground.

The short trail to Horse Trough Falls lies at the very head of the campground. The trail leads 0.1 mile to a viewing platform that looks up at the falls. The cascade expands from 2 to more than 30 feet before it gathers again to flow into the Chattahoochee River, just above the campground.

:: Ratings

BEAUTY: ★ ★ ★ ★
PRIVACY: ★ ★ ★
SPACIOUSNESS: ★ ★ ★ ★ ★
QUIET: ★ ★ ★ ★ ★
SECURITY: ★ ★ ★ ★
CLEANLINESS: ★ ★ ★ ★

:: Key Information

ADDRESS: P.O. Box 196, Burton Rd., Clarkesville, GA 30523

OPERATED BY: U.S. Forest Service

CONTACT: 706-754-6221; www.fs.usda.gov/conf

OPEN: Mid-march–October

SITES: 34

SITE AMENITIES: Tent pad, fire grate, lantern post, picnic table

ASSIGNMENT: First come, first served

REGISTRATION: Self-registration on-site

FACILITIES: Hand-pumped water, flush toilets

PARKING: At campsites

FEE: $12

ELEVATION: 2,100 feet

RESTRICTIONS
- **Pets:** On leash only
- **Fires:** In fire rings only
- **Alcohol:** At campsites only
- **Vehicles:** 22-foot trailer length limit
- **Other:** 14-day stay limit

Another popular hike is the 1.6-mile tramp to Poplar Stomp Gap and the Appalachian Trail on old FR 44-C. Once on the AT, turn left and hike to the Low Gap shelter, passing a mature hardwood forest en route. Mountain bikers will like the 7-mile loop ride around the Jasus Creek watershed. The loop starts 4.6 miles below the campground on gated FR 44-C.

The Chattahoochee River and its many tributaries offer abundant trout fishing. Low Gap Branch and Jasus Creek provide the angler with miles of remote wilderness, where you can fish far back in thick forest that is normally trampled only by the wild creatures of the Mark Trail Wilderness.

The highlight of my Upper Chattahoochee River adventure was the 38-mile loop drive along the Russel–Brasstown Scenic Byway that is formed by highways 17, 180, 348, and 356. First, I drove out FR 44 to US 129 over Unicoi Gap and then north to the High Shoals Scenic Area. I hiked a mile to the falls—a series of five drops totaling 300 feet. Afterward, I drove to Brasstown Bald,

Georgia's highest point. I took the half-mile walk to the viewing tower at 4,784 feet. There I was treated to a 360-degree view of the surrounding mountains.

On I drove, along streams and on top of ridges, taking in the scenery. I stopped at Dukes Creek Falls, a 150-foot drop down a sheer granite canyon. Beyond the town of Helen was Anna Ruby Falls. It is a double falls, 0.4 miles from the trailhead at the confluence of Curtis and York creeks. I then returned to the Upper Chattahoochee Campground thinking that maybe the byway should be called the Falls Byway.

That evening, the skies were clear, so after supper I decided to sleep out in the open. Later, I felt a pitter-patter on my face and groggily erected my shelter just in time for a major downpour. The next morning, the Chattahoochee River was roaring beside my camp. I returned to Horse Trough Falls to see a crashing display of whitewater that wasn't present the day before. As I drove out of the campground that morning, I felt extremely satisfied with my experience. You will, too.

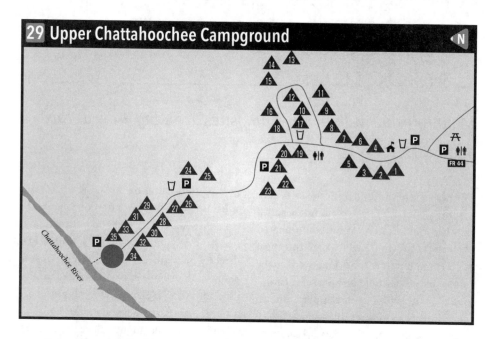

:: Getting There

From Cleveland, take GA 75 North 17 miles. Turn left on FR 44 and continue 5 miles. Upper Chattahoochee Campground will be on your right.

GPS COORDINATES   N34° 47' 20.07"   W83° 46' 53.83"

30

Vogel State Park Campground

Mountainside walk-in tent campsites are a big draw at this state park.

This is the second oldest state park in Georgia. Located amid Chattahoochee National Forest on land donated by Fred Vogel, the park makes the most of its mountain environs. One look at the campground will tell you that. The campground is great for tent campers, due to the 18 walk-in campsites, plus a loop exclusively for tents, vans, and pop-up campers. Hikers love to tackle the trails that traverse the mountains; when they return to their campsite, they still feel at one with nature, as the campground is integrated into the sylvan scenery.

Pass the plethora of cabins to enter the campground, located in the Wolf Creek drainage area. The rich forest overhead is a mixture of Appalachian hardwoods and fragrant white pines. Cross the bridge over Burnett Branch. The lower sites, 1–31, aren't worth fooling with, as the too-close sites are the domain of the big rigs. Come to the main walk-in tent-camping area, sites A–P. The forest is thick and lush overhead in the tent-camping area. Most of the sites are first rate in situation and location. Site A is the closest and almost qualifies as a drive-up site. Sites B and C are directly on Wolf Creek and require just a short walk. An upper parking area is available for sites D–H. Site D is all alone on a hill so steep that a wooden tent pad was added for a good night's sleep. Sites E–H are located along a trail heading up a rocky slope that defines the word mountain. Fear not, the sites have been leveled and the rocks removed at each immediate camping area. Sites G and H are of special note for solitude lovers and those that don't mind earning their great spot.

A third parking area is situated for sites I–L. These are all good sites. Head up a richly wooded hillside and reach L first. It is set along a small streamlet bordered by mountain laurel. The sites get better as you climb the hill, culminating in site I. The last parking area is for sites M–P. These are the least desirable of the walk-in sites but are close to the bathhouse that serves the area.

Return to the main camping area and discount sites 32–37. Turn left onto the loop with sites 62–85. This is the loop for tents, vans, and pop-ups. The narrow road is curvy and offers sites carved into the landscape. Some are hillside sites; others are in flats. This loop has mostly good sites, though a few are too close together. A bathhouse is on

:: Ratings

BEAUTY: ★ ★ ★ ★
PRIVACY: ★ ★ ★ ★
SPACIOUSNESS: ★ ★ ★
QUIET: ★ ★ ★
SECURITY: ★ ★ ★ ★ ★
CLEANLINESS: ★ ★ ★ ★

:: Key Information

ADDRESS: 7845 Vogel State Park Rd., Blairsville, GA 30512

OPERATED BY: Georgia State Parks

CONTACT: 706-745-2628, **gastateparks .org**; reservations 800-864-7275

OPEN: Year-round

SITES: 18 walk-in, 85 others

SITE AMENITIES: Walk-in tent sites have picnic table, fire ring, tent pad, lantern post, upright grill; others also have water and electricity

ASSIGNMENT: First come, first served or by reservation

REGISTRATION: At park office

FACILITIES: Hot showers, flush toilets

PARKING: At walk-in tent parking and at campsites

FEE: $20 walk-in, $27–$30 others

ELEVATION: 2,300 feet

RESTRICTIONS
- **Pets:** On leash only
- **Fires:** In fire rings only
- **Alcohol:** At campsites only
- **Vehicles:** 2 vehicles per site
- **Other:** 14-day stay limit

the upper end of the loop. The last camping area is along a road bordering Wolf Creek. All streamside sites are good and enjoy the creek resonating nearby. They are coveted by big rigs and tenters alike. Two walk-in sites are at the head of the loop. Campsite Q is on a hill and has great solitude. Campsite R is on a bluff overlooking Wolf Creek and would be a treat on a hot day, as it is well shaded. The campground fills on nice spring and fall weekends, and just about every weekend during summer. Reservations are highly recommended.

Activities at the park are plentiful. Watery action is centered on Lake Trahlyta, named for a Cherokee princess. This mountain impoundment offers a swim beach and paddle boats for tooling around the lake, or fishing for trout in spring and bass or bream in summer. The new Civilian Conservation Corps Museum is located near the lake and details the story of the young men who developed this park during the Great Depression. A miniature golf course is adjacent to the park office.

Despite the above attractions, this is a hiker's park. Even the least walking-inclined need to venture on the Byron Reese Nature Trail. Here, you can see more than 20 species of trees that grow within this state park. See the cascade on the Trahlyta Falls Spur Trail. The Bear Hair Gap Trail makes a 3.9-mile loop. It features an overlook where you can gaze down on Lake Trahlyta and the mountains beyond. You can also enjoy many different mountain environments that feature the flora of Southern Appalachia in all their glory. Start early, and pack lunch and water if you want to tackle the Coosa Backcountry Trail as a day hiker. It makes a 13-plus-mile loop and is used by backpackers for overnight trips. This hike takes on such places as Slaughter Mountain, Coosa Bald, and Wildcat Knob, in addition to crossing streams too. If you want to learn more about the area without all the walking, a park naturalist hosts enrichment programs five days a week during summer, which offer a good way to learn about the botanically rich park, Georgia's second-oldest protected area.

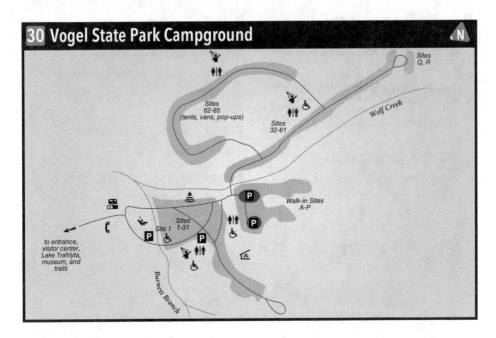

:: Getting There

From Dahlonega, follow US 19 North 25 miles to the state park.

GPS COORDINATES   N34° 46' 12.25"   W83° 55' 5.08"

31

War Hill Campground

This small campground is nearly encircled by water.

The **name** of this relaxing lakeside camping destination—War Hill—contrasts mightily with the realities of this campground located on the Chestatee River arm of Lake Lanier. Your only battles will likely be finding a campsite during ideal weather summer weekends in this small campground. Or maybe getting your camping buddy to make a water run to the spigot atop the hill, or avoiding the last hamburger that sat on the grill a few minutes too long. Name aside, War Hill offers a relatively less hectic setting than the southern shores of Lake Lanier. My spring weekend visit was quiet, but, in full disclosure, a big storm was headed our way. The only other group at War Hill was in the same predicament as me, trying to batten down the hatches as a powerful wind was threatening to blow down tents and blow away just about everything on the picnic table and anything else that wasn't nailed down. The winds were whipping off Lake Lanier, and I was glad this part of the lake isn't near the open water (as lower stretches near Buford Dam are). In that case, we could've roped ourselves to the tent and just flown back home. That evening, the wind died and the rain followed, long after we had bedded down, not interrupting our evening cookout.

The campground is on a hill nearly encircled by water and connected to the mainland by a narrow peninsula. Pass the campground host, who staffs the area and helps keep War Hill safe and secure. The park road reaches War Hill. Begin a loop around the hill, first passing an attractive picnic area on your right to reach the camping area. A mix of pines and hardwoods shades the well-manicured camping areas. Site 1 is a pull-through site. The main camping area is down the hill by the water. Steps lead down to the site. Site 2 is directly on the water at a point. Many steps lead down to this campsite as well. The next set of sites are located a good distance down the road. Reach site 3, which is one of only two campsites not directly on the water. Site 4 is the shadiest site in the campground, as a pine thicket keeps the sun away. Sites 5–8 are a little close together but are all on the water. Curve around to site 9, which is on the water and offers much better solitude. Site 10 is the second site inside the loop and isn't bad, other than not being on the water. This is a water lover's campground.

Curve along and reach more good waterside sites. Site 11 looks across the water at another Army Corps of Engineers Campground, Boling Mill, which is much larger and busier than War Hill. War Hill will fill on summer holiday weekends and nice summer weekends. Site 12 is large and may be

:: Ratings

BEAUTY: ★ ★ ★ ★
PRIVACY: ★ ★ ★
SPACIOUSNESS: ★ ★ ★ ★
QUIET: ★ ★ ★
SECURITY: ★ ★ ★ ★
CLEANLINESS: ★ ★ ★ ★

:: Key Information

ADDRESS: 7800 Shadburn Ferry Rd., Cumming, GA 30041

OPERATED BY: U.S. Army Corps of Engineers

CONTACT: 770-945-9531, **www.sam .usace.army.mil/Missions/CivilWorks /Recreation/LakeSidneyLanier**

OPEN: First weekend in April through the first weekend in September

SITES: 14

SITE AMENITIES: Picnic table, fire grate, upright grill, lantern post, tent pad

ASSIGNMENT: First come, first served

REGISTRATION: Self-registration on-site

FACILITIES: Water spigots, flush toilets

PARKING: At campsites only

FEE: $22

ELEVATION: 1,100 feet

RESTRICTIONS
- **Pets:** On leash only
- **Fires:** In fire rings only
- **Alcohol:** Prohibited
- **Vehicles:** 3 vehicles per campsite
- **Other:** 14-day stay limit

the prettiest campsite of them all. Site 13 is well shaded and has ample solitude. Site 14 requires a walk down to the water but overlooks a cove adjacent to War Hill. A restroom with flush toilets is located on a short road between site 14 and the picnic area. The campground water spigot is up here too.

Many campers like to pull their boats directly up to their campsites. However, War Hill does have a big boat ramp. Here, you can access the water to indulge in your favorite aquatic activity, whether it be boating, fishing, or skiing. Narrow arms and islands characterize this part of the lake. Be apprised that even this part of Lake Lanier can hop

during high summer weekends. There is no completely escaping the hustle and bustle on this lake. Nevertheless, this area is less busy than locales down south. A long and wide swim beach is located between the boat ramp and the campground. The area is somewhat protected by being in a cove. Pines shade green grass that lines the swim beach. Floating buoys delineate the swim area. A super-long pier extends outward from the cove and is good for fishing or just relaxing by the water. However, you don't need the pier to relax by the water, as you can do that at your campsite on War Hill, in spite of its decidedly unrelaxing name.

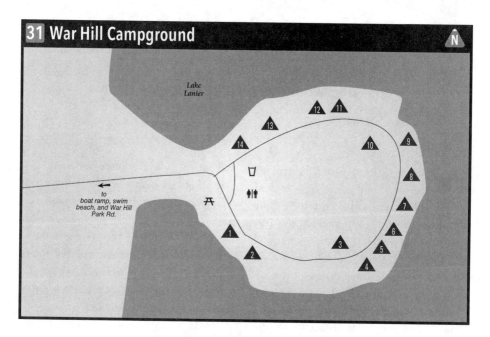

31 War Hill Campground

Lake Lanier

to
boat ramp, swim
beach, and War Hill
Park Rd.

:: Getting There

From the junction of GA 400 and GA 53 east of Dawsonville, head east on GA 53 1.8 miles to War Hill Park Road. Turn left on War Hill Park Road and follow it 4 miles to reach the recreation area.

GPS COORDINATES   N34° 20' 3.48"   W83° 57' 47.42"

32

Wildcat Campground

Wildlife, water, and wilderness are only a trail away at Wildcat Campground.

Wildcat **Campground** is actually two rough and rustic areas located in the 12,600-acre Lake Burton Wildlife Management Area, contiguous to the Tray Mountain Wilderness. A single-lane road with turnouts traces Wildcat Creek and all but eliminates RVs from entering the area. The Forest Service banished roadside camping along Wildcat Creek and constructed these campgrounds to concentrate the impact of human visitors in two areas. The Lake Burton Wildlife Management Area is lightly used except during hunting season.

The two campgrounds are spartan and will put you in the mood for outdoor recreation. Both areas have vault flush toilets and recycling bins. You must get your water from the creek. Be sure to treat or boil it before consuming. Or better yet, bring your own.

Wildcat Area 1 is located just above the confluence of Wildcat Creek and Jessie Branch. Most of the 16 sites are pinched on either side of a loop road circling a creekside flat. However, a few sites rest outside the loop and require a short

:: Ratings

BEAUTY: ★ ★ ★ ★
PRIVACY: ★ ★ ★
SPACIOUSNESS: ★ ★ ★
QUIET: ★ ★ ★ ★
SECURITY: ★ ★ ★
CLEANLINESS: ★ ★ ★ ★

walk uphill, offering more seclusion and space. Big trees are scattered around the campground, providing ample shade and making up for minimal groundcover. An interesting feature of the campground is the abundance of large rocks placed about the campground by the Forest Service for aesthetics and site delineation. They also make good seats and great tables.

Wildcat Area 2 is bigger and, in my opinion, the better of the two. It has 16 campsites arranged along a figure-eight creekside loop. Large rocks are even more abundant here beneath the tall forest. In addition, the sites here are larger than at Wildcat Area 1. A grassy field created by the Forest Service as a wildlife opening is adjacent to the campground, providing a good escape should you feel closed in by the forest. Just across the creek is the Tray Mountain Wilderness boundary.

For water fun, try fishing, swimming, and boating. Wildcat Creek is stocked weekly during the summer with trout from the Lake Burton Hatchery. FR 26 provides easy access to good pools, as well as the Sliding Rock, a popular swimming hole where you can skim over a slippery rock into a cool mountain stream. Be careful, though; those rocks are slippery. The slide is visible from FR 26 before you reach the campgrounds. For true backwoods fishing, follow Wildcat Creek into the wilderness and away from the road. Nearby Lake Burton provides other

:: Key Information

ADDRESS: 825 US 441, Clayton, GA 30525

OPERATED BY: U.S. Forest Service

CONTACT: 706-782-3320, www.fs.usda.gov/conf

OPEN: Year-round

SITES: Area 1, 16; Area 2, 16

SITE AMENITIES: Tent pad, lantern post, fire pit, picnic table

ASSIGNMENT: First come, first served

REGISTRATION: Self-registration on-site

FACILITIES: Vault toilets

PARKING: At campsites only

FEE: $10

ELEVATION: Area 1, 2,100 feet; Area 2, 2,400 feet

RESTRICTIONS
- **Pets:** On leash only
- **Fires:** In fire rings only
- **Alcohol:** At campsites only
- **Vehicles:** 22-foot trailer length limit
- **Other:** 14-day stay limit

watery recreation opportunities if you own (or want to rent) a boat.

No trails start from the campgrounds, but you'll find plenty nearby. Just up FR 26 are the Bramlett Ridge and Pigpen Ridge trails. Bramlett Ridge Trail leads 2 miles into the heart of the Tray Mountain Wilderness, intersecting the Appalachian Trail at Round Top. Follow the AT north and you can loop back to your car from Addis Gap. The Pigpen Ridge Trail leads east 2 miles to Moccasin Creek and a series of waterfalls and slides. You can also access the Moccasin Creek Trail from Moccasin Creek State Park at Lake Burton.

Moccasin Creek is a gem of a trail. It combines scenic beauty with wildlife openings, enabling you to see the Forest Service's efforts to create a better habitat for the region's fauna. Wildlife openings are man-made clearings containing highly nutritional plants and grasses that are sown for

birds, turkey, deer, and other animals. Forest and grassland interface in these openings, producing "edges" where a greater variety of food plants from both environments mix to attract wildlife. Wildlife management is a key element of the Forest Service's multiple-use concept for our national forests.

Other trails with wildlife openings, such as North Fork Trail, Parks Gap Trail, and old Deep Gap Road, connect with the Moccasin Creek Trail to form wildlife viewing loops. The side trails are rarely used during the summer and can provide an isolated wildlife hiking experience. Get the Lake Burton Wildlife Management Area map from the Moccasin Creek State Park office.

Kastner's Store is located just south of FR 26 on GA 197 if you need supplies. Other services can be accessed along this road as well. Wildcat is an appropriate name for this campground in the middle of a wildlife management area.

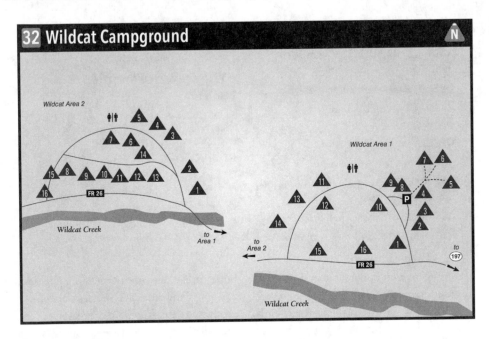

:: Getting There

Take GA 197 North from Clarkesville 22 miles. Turn left up a steep hill on FR 26. Follow FR 26 3 miles to Wildcat Camping Area 1; it will be on your right. Wildcat Camping Area 2 is 1 mile farther, also on your right.

GPS COORDINATES   N34° 49' 36.80"   W83° 37' 5.44"

Middle Georgia

33

Bussey Point Campground

This campground on a peninsula offers waterfront campsites as well as land and water recreation.

Bussey Point is the best choice on Strom Thurmond Lake for pure tent campers. South Carolina and Georgia share Thurmond Lake. In Georgia, the lake is sometimes referred to as Clarks Hill Lake, so don't let the name confuse you. Name aside, Bussey Point is the most prominent peninsula on this very large lake. As such, it is surrounded on three sides by water, at the tip where the Little River arm and Savannah River arm of the lake meet. The pretty camping area is located on a small peninsula of its own, a subpeninsula of the primary Bussey Point peninsula. The campground can be your base camp for enjoying all the lake has to offer, as well as the large, wild, and wooded Bussey Point via trails that course through it.

Each campsite here is good quality and lakefront. Landscaping timbers have been added to delineate and level the campsites. Pass the fee station and trail to the pump well, then curve to the lake. Reach sites 1 and 2, which share a common spur road but then split apart. Site 1 is directly on the water yet shaded by oaks, pines, cedars, hickories, and other hardwoods. A thick brushy understory divides the sites. Site 2 is a bit off the water but well shaded. A second road leads to sites 3 and 4, both well-shaded, well-separated, waterfront sites.

A small road joins sites 5 and 6. These sites are large and more open. Site 7 is elevated a bit and overlooks the water and an island in the distance. Site 8 offers yet another lakefront site. Site 9 has a small spur road of its own. Site 10 is at the end of the line, just before an auto turnaround. A vault toilet is located over here, so folks accessing the trail system, which starts just over a short bridge from the auto turnaround, use it, as well as fellow campers. The pump well can be accessed by trail near the fee station or by driving around toward the area boat ramp. Look for the pump well on the left before you reach the boat ramp.

I visited during a spring weekday and was the only camper. The dogwoods brightened the forest with their blooms, the lake was at full pool, and it seemed the forest was greening and growing before my very eyes. Despite the solitude during my visit, spring weekends are the most popular time for this overlooked camping area. You should be able to get a site here any other time, weekend or weekday, despite it having only 10 campsites.

Bussey Point primitive area, the main peninsula, has trails aplenty to keep hikers, equestrians, and mountain bikers busy. The trailhead is just a short walk from the

:: Ratings

BEAUTY: ★ ★ ★ ★
PRIVACY: ★ ★ ★ ★
SPACIOUSNESS: ★ ★ ★ ★
QUIET: ★ ★ ★
SECURITY: ★ ★ ★
CLEANLINESS: ★ ★ ★

:: Key Information

ADDRESS: Route 1, Box 6, Clarks Hill, SC 29821

OPERATED BY: U.S. Army Corps of Engineers

CONTACT: 800-533-3478, **www.sas .usace.army.mil/About/Divisionsand Offices/OperationsDivision/JStrom ThurmondDamandLake**

OPEN: Year-round

SITES: 10

SITE AMENITIES: Picnic table, fire ring, lantern post, tent pad, garbage can

ASSIGNMENT: First come, first served

REGISTRATION: No registration

FACILITIES: Pump well, vault toilets

PARKING: At campsites only

FEE: $6

ELEVATION: 340 feet

RESTRICTIONS
- **Pets:** On leash only
- **Fires:** In fire rings only
- **Alcohol:** At campsites only
- **Vehicles:** None
- **Other:** 14-day stay limit

campground. These paths, mostly old roads, reach out to all fingers of the peninsula. Food plots have been established in places to enhance wildlife out here—primarily deer and turkeys. The trails system has several highlights, including an observation tower where you can look over the land and lake, a lakeside picnic area, and a shelter. Your best bet for exploring these trails is to call ahead and ask for a trail map.

Despite the trails, water recreation—whether it be fishing, boating, waterskiing, or swimming—is the biggest draw. Campers swim and fish from the day-use area near campsite 10, as well as the boat ramp located on a side road away from the campground. Once you hit the water, you'll see that Lake Thurmond is a huge recreation destination. Completed in 1954, the lake now hosts 7 million visitors annually. But it doesn't seem that way at Bussey Point, the least used campground on the Georgia side of the lake. Therefore, a tent camper can find a little solitude along these 1,200 miles of shoreline, drainages of the Savannah and Little rivers. The lake also has more than 100 islands that add a scenic touch to the impoundment. It might seem that the lake also has 100 campgrounds, but you'll likely find that Bussey Point offers the best pure tent-camping experience on this side of Thurmond Lake.

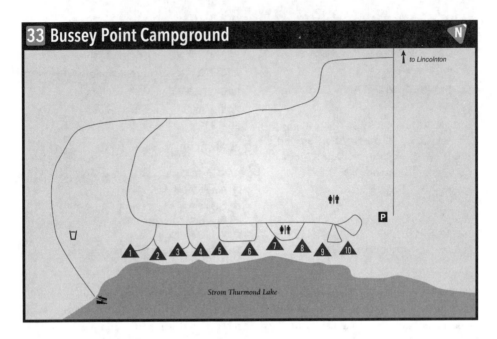

33 Bussey Point Campground

to Lincolnton

P

Strom Thurmond Lake

:: Getting There

From Lincolnton, take GA 47 South 6 miles to GA 220. Take a left onto GA 220 East and follow it 2 miles to Double Branch Road. Turn right and follow Double Branch Road to dead-end at the campground after 5.3 miles.

GPS COORDINATES   N33° 42' 14.18"   W82° 15' 35.87"

34

F. D. Roosevelt State Park Campground

Georgia's largest state park is also big on recreation opportunities.

F. **D. Roosevelt State Park's** boasts are many: It is Georgia's largest state park and most historic in terms of its development because its construction was personally supervised by America's longest-serving president, Franklin Delano Roosevelt. The park, to some, has the best hiking in the state park system, with 23-mile Pine Mountain Trail the linchpin in the other 14 miles of trails. It has a spring-fed stone swimming pool, scenic drive, and is only 11 miles distant from FDR's Little White House in Warm Springs, Georgia.

Warm Springs first attracted the president to the area while he was seeking relief from polio, which he had contracted in 1921. During his travels to Georgia seeking a cure, he discovered the beauty of this area, which ultimately led Pine Mountain to be developed as a state park. Today, it is one of Georgia's best destinations, including a campground that will suit your needs.

:: Ratings

BEAUTY: ★ ★ ★
PRIVACY: ★ ★ ★
SPACIOUSNESS: ★ ★ ★
QUIET: ★ ★ ★
SECURITY: ★ ★ ★ ★
CLEANLINESS: ★ ★ ★ ★

The campground is situated on the shore of Lake Delanor. Reach Lower Camping Area 1 first as you enter the campground from the park office. Typical of the five camping areas here, it has some fine sites and some real dogs. Check out the narrow road closest to the lake. The sites have been leveled and look directly over the water. I enjoyed staying in site 108. Next, reach Camping Area 2. It has large sites delineated with landscaping timbers beneath a shady forest of pines and hardwoods, but it is the domain of the big rigs. Camping Area 3 loops up a hollow and has large, quiet sites that are good for tent campers. Camping Area 4 is set on a ridgeline. The sites are smaller and don't have parking pads, making them de facto tent sites. They are heavily shaded and off the beaten path. The road slopes down a hollow to other quiet sites. Camping Area 5 is on the "back 40" of the campground, away from the hubbub. It is the most level loop and has a mix of bad, okay, and good campsites. Generally, the sites on Loop 5 are larger than most, and several are well shaded too. The last locale is Upper Camping Area 6. It has rougher sites behind the camp store. Some are a little too close to the camp store, but the narrow, winding gravel road repels RVs.

Your best bet for finding a good site is to diligently drive around and inspect the campground, as Georgia state parks don't

:: Key Information

ADDRESS: 2970 GA 190, Pine Mountain, GA 31822	**REGISTRATION:** At park office
OPERATED BY: Georgia State Parks	**FACILITIES:** Hot showers, flush toilets, laundry, picnic shelters, camp store
CONTACT: 706-663-4858, gastateparks.org; reservations 800-864-7275	**PARKING:** At campsites only
	FEE: $28
OPEN: Year-round	**ELEVATION:** 900 feet
SITES: 109	
SITE AMENITIES: Picnic table, fire ring, tent pad, water, electricity	**RESTRICTIONS**
ASSIGNMENT: First come, first served and by reservation	■ **Pets:** On leash only
	■ **Fires:** In fire rings only
	■ **Alcohol:** At campsites only
	■ **Vehicles:** 2 vehicles per site
	■ **Other:** 14-day stay limit

allow specific site reservations. The park campground will fill most every weekend of the year, except for the weekends of January and February. Reservations are highly recommended. Note that areas 2 and 4 are always open. The others are open as needed, which means on weekends and nearly every day in summer. Covered picnic shelters are dispersed throughout the campground and make for a dry place to hang out during rainy times.

A concessionaire leads guided horseback rides through the park if you don't feel like hiking but still want to explore. Hiking is as easy as walking from your tent. The Delano Trail roughly circles the campground, and the Mountain Creek Nature Trail actually starts at the campground. Another path leads to the stone swimming pool down by GA 354. The Pine Mountain Trail is the master path of the park. Several loop hikes can be made using the Pine Mountain Trail in conjunction with other spur trails. The Wolfden Loop travels 6.7 miles and boasts of having one of the most beautiful trail stretches in the Southeast. The Overlook Loop, 3.4 miles in length, is the newest loop in the trail system.

Make a scenic drive through the park in conjunction with a visit to the Little White House, where you can also see the unfinished portrait of Roosevelt and learn the story behind the painting. The Dowdell Knob Loop can be hiked in conjunction with a scenic drive along the crest of Pine Mountain. Dowdell Knob was one of FDR's favorite vista spots. Here, you can picnic where he did, enjoy the views, and go on a hike. And when you return home, you will be the one boasting about this star of the Georgia state park system.

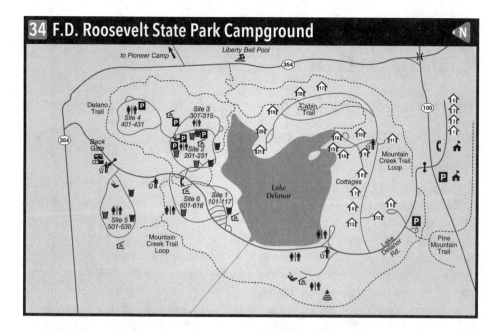

:: Getting There

From Exit 42 on I-185, head south on US 27 11 miles, passing through the town of Pine Mountain at mile 10. One mile beyond Pine Mountain, turn left onto GA 354 East and follow it 2.5 miles to GA 190. Turn right here and reach the park office shortly, on your left.

GPS COORDINATES   N32° 50' 33.14"   W84° 49' 43.71"

35

George L. Smith State Park Campground

The cypress-studded lake here is a sight to see, and you can view it from the many lakeside campsites.

Have you ever seen a cypress-lined lake? Well, this isn't one of them. This lake has moss-draped cypress trees not only around the lake but also throughout the lake. Luckily for lake explorers, the park has three marked boat trails coursing among the 412-acre impoundment, backed up from a gristmill from the 1800s. "Brooding swamp" is a clichéd term, but it is hard to otherwise describe just what you'll see out here. Just be glad the boat trails are out here—otherwise "two turns of a boat can get you lost," as it was explained to me. The aforementioned mill, which also acts as a dam and covered bridge, is a historic site and an added bonus of visiting this watery park with a small, attractive, but busy campground.

The campground is laid out in a loop sloping down toward George L. Smith Lake. Pine trees populate the loop center, which also has a grassy play area and a bathhouse. Cruise past some pull-through RV sites, then begin the pull-up lakeside campsites. Hardwoods and some pines provide maximum shade. Heavy vegetation screens sites from one another. The sites are just a few feet away from and a few feet above the cypress-laden waters. Landscaping timbers keep the sites level. Many sites are two-tiered. Deft paddlers will be able to pull their boats directly to the campsites amid the hundreds of trees growing out of the water. Fourteen sites run along the lake before reaching two almost connected sites, with only one lakeside. Then the desirable sites resume, with five more camps along the lake. The last couple of lakeside sites are a little higher and have steps leading down to the water. A few more pull-through sites are on the inside of the loop.

George L. Smith State Park has only 25 sites, and these are coveted. This place will fill every weekend from spring through fall. Reservations are highly recommended. Many visitors come from Savannah seeking a change of scenery. Actually, just about anybody coming from anywhere will be seeing something different here than what they see at home. This tree-filled lake is scenic!

And the lake is definitely the attraction here. One of two boat launches is located conveniently near the campground. If you don't have your own boat, rent a canoe or johnboat from the park by the hour or by the day. They also rent electric motors. There's a 10-horsepower limit if you have your own

:: Ratings

BEAUTY: ★ ★ ★
PRIVACY: ★ ★ ★
SPACIOUSNESS: ★ ★ ★
QUIET: ★ ★ ★ ★
SECURITY: ★ ★ ★
CLEANLINESS: ★ ★ ★ ★

:: Key Information

ADDRESS: 371 George L. Smith State Park Rd., Twin City, GA 30471

OPERATED BY: Georgia State Parks

CONTACT: 478-763-2759, **gastateparks.org;** reservations 800-864-7275

OPEN: Year-round

SITES: 25

SITE AMENITIES: Picnic table, fire ring, tent pad, lantern post, water, electricity

ASSIGNMENT: First come, first served and by reservation

REGISTRATION: At park office

FACILITIES: Hot showers, flush toilets, laundry, phone

PARKING: At campsites only

FEE: $28

ELEVATION: 220 feet

RESTRICTIONS
- **Pets:** On leash only
- **Fires:** In fire rings only
- **Alcohol:** At campsites only
- **Vehicles:** 2 vehicles per site
- **Other:** 14-day stay limit

motor, but once you see the lake you'll wonder where there is enough open water to get a head of steam. This park is growing in popularity with paddlers. Canoers and kayakers explore among the cypress trees, both to fish and just to sightsee. Bring your camera. Largemouth bass can be caught year-round, crappie when it's cooler, and bream when it warms up. Each of the boat trails exceeds 4 miles in length. The Red Trail runs up the middle of the long lake. The Yellow Trail heads along the western shoreline, and the Blue Trail keeps along the eastern bank. All trails meet on the north end of the 120-plus-year-old impoundment.

You can get your shoes dirty walking around some of the land trails on the park. The Deer Run Hiking Trail travels in a sand ridge ecosystem for 3 miles. Gopher tortoises like it up here. More trails leave from the boat dock on the west shore, by the new cabins. The Squirrel Run Trail connects the campground to the park office and Mill House. The Brown Thrasher Trail makes a short loop behind the old park cabins.

It's only a couple of yards' walk from the park office to the Mill House. Built in 1880, this structure has about everything rolled into one. The Mill House started out as a dam, with floodgates to create water power to turn a turbine and then power all kinds of things. It was a sawmill to cut timber for the covered bridge and saw lumber for area residents. It was a gristmill for grinding corn. It has even bailed cotton. The whole thing is original except for the floor, and the gristmill is still in working order.

Pass through the covered bridge to pick up the Deer Run Hiking Trail. Anglers can often be seen bank fishing below the mill dam. The Mill House area has a certain quaintness to it. And it complements the park lake, which offers some serious scenery of its own.

35 George L. Smith State Park Campground

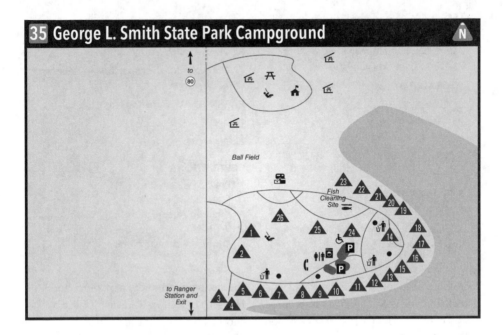

:: Getting There

From Exit 104 on I-16, take GA 23 North 13 miles to George L. Smith State Park Road, passing through downtown Metter on the way. Turn right on George L. Smith State Park Road and follow it to enter the park.

GPS COORDINATES N32° 32' 41.17" W82° 07' 3.23"

36

Hesters Ferry Campground

Hesters Ferry stakes the claim as the prettiest campground on Strom Thurmond Lake.

Retired seniors generally staff the developed Army Corps of Engineers campgrounds. They work the campground entrance station, register campers, and answer questions, including those from persistent outdoor writers. On my visit to Hesters Ferry, the campground host told me flatly that this was the most attractive campground on Strom Thurmond Lake (also known as Clarks Hill Lake). After looking around, I could see her point. It is set on the peninsula between the Newford Creek arm and Fishing Creek arm of the lake. The hilly woods and waterfront campsites combine to make for wooded getaways that offer great views into the dammed Savannah River.

The campground is divided into two distinct and widely separated loops. The first loop has sites 1–16. A beautiful forest of pine, cedar, maple, dogwood, sweet gum, and oaks adds a scenic touch to the hilly terrain. Heavy brush divides the sites. Sites 1–4 are on a small cove. These sites, like all the others, are waterfront. Site 5 is large. Site 6 is shaded. Sites 7 and 8 are on a short spur

road, with site 8 being directly on a point and highly coveted. Sites 9 and 10 are on the water. The campground bathhouse is across from site 10. Sites 11–16 are on a low bluff overlooking the water, but the lake is a little harder to access from here. These sites are well shaded, however. Sites 15 and 16 offer good solitude. The campsites on this first loop all have water and electricity but are recommended nonetheless.

The second loop is on a point with sites 17–26. There is no water and electricity here, leaving this as the sole domain of the tents. Sites 17 and 18 are a bit close together, but both are waterfront on a cove. Dip past a hollow, then come to sites 19 and 20, which are close to the water. Sites 21 and 22 offer good lake views. Sites 23 and 24 overlook the bulk of the lake. Site 25, on a point, is the most desired site in the whole campground and, according to the campground host, the best site at Hesters Ferry. Site 26 doesn't have quite the view, but only compared to site 25. The sites are well spaced from one another. A vault toilet serves this loop, leaving campers to visit the other loop for showering. You must also go to the other loop to get your water.

With a mere 26 sites, the campground can only get so busy. Most campgrounds with reservable sites are much larger, so here you get to reserve sites with the safety and convenience of a campground host without feeling like you are in "Campgroundtown."

:: Ratings

BEAUTY: ★ ★ ★ ★
PRIVACY: ★ ★ ★ ★
SPACIOUSNESS: ★ ★ ★ ★
QUIET: ★ ★ ★
SECURITY: ★ ★ ★ ★ ★
CLEANLINESS: ★ ★ ★ ★

:: Key Information

ADDRESS: Route 1, Box 12, Clarks Hill, SC 29821	**ASSIGNMENT:** First come, first served and by reservation
OPERATED BY: U.S. Army Corps of Engineers	**REGISTRATION:** At campground entrance station
CONTACT: 800-533-3478, **www.sas .usace.army.mil/About/Divisionsand Offices/OperationsDivision/JStrom ThurmondDamandLake;** reservations 877-444-6777, **recreation.gov**	**FACILITIES:** Hot showers, flush toilets
	PARKING: At campsites only
	FEE: $18 tent, $22 water and electric
	ELEVATION: 340 feet
OPEN: April–September	**RESTRICTIONS**
SITES: 10 tent, 16 water and electric	■ **Pets:** On leash only
SITE AMENITIES: Picnic table, fire ring, lantern post, tent pad, food prep table, upright grill	■ **Fires:** In fire rings only
	■ **Alcohol:** At campsites only
	■ **Vehicles:** All vehicles must be on campsite or driveway
	■ **Other:** 14-day stay limit

On nice summer weekends and summer weekend holidays, Hesters Ferry will have a full house. Reservations are recommended. All campsites except 17 and 18 are reservable.

This is a relaxed campground where families and friends congregate together. The Army Corps of Engineers must have anticipated that campers here like to eat because they've added a food preparation table and upright grill to all the campsites. By the way, it's a long way to stores from here, so bring all your food and supplies; otherwise, you'll be running the roads instead of sitting in the shade.

There is no formal swim beach here. Most campers just swim along the shoreline from their campsites. The paved campground road is wide and relatively unused, making for good casual bicycling. Boating, both motorized and self-propelled, is popular here. A boat ramp is near the first loop. Fishing is popular too. Some claim the Fishing Creek arm to have the best fishing on the whole lake—it wasn't named Fishing Creek for nothing. Even if you don't fish, you will come back from Hesters Ferry agreeing that this is the prettiest campground on Strom Thurmond Lake.

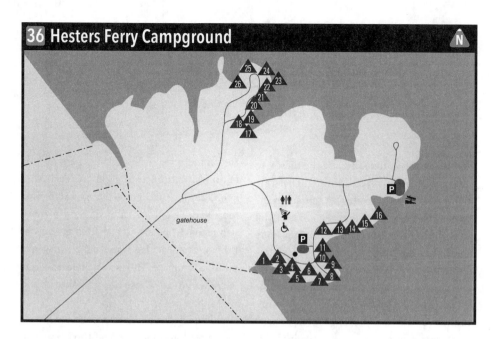

36 Hesters Ferry Campground

gatehouse

:: Getting There

From Washington, keep east on GA 44 17 miles to GA 79 and a four-way stop. GA 44 ends here. However, keep forward through the four-way stop, now on Graball Road, continuing 2.6 miles, then veer left onto the signed gravel road to enter the campground.

GPS COORDINATES   N33° 56' 20.52"   W82° 32' 14.42"

37

Holiday Campground

This well-kept campground has walk-in tent sites directly on West Point Lake.

The walk-in tent sites are the reason to come here, plain and simple. These are among the best campsites for tenters in the state of Georgia. They are so good that you may not want to leave your site. And there aren't just a few of them tossed in as an after-thought—there are a whopping 35 walk-in tent sites. That means no matter what time of year, save for summer holiday weekends, you will be able to get a first-rate campsite overlooking west Georgia's West Point Lake. And if you want a drive-up campsite, 16 of them are nonelectric and also offer lakefront vistas. Furthermore, this is a well-designed, spare-no-expense Army Corps of Engineers campground, where even the electric sites aren't bad. Recreation opportunities are centered on West Point Lake, plus a little hiking and biking, which can also be enjoyed directly from the campground.

You will definitely need a map to get around this large campground, spread far and wide over a peninsula jutting into West Point Lake. There are so many loops at different sites that I am only going to describe the nonelectric sites. After passing the entrance station, turn right to reach sites 5–9. They are on their own large and private loop with lakefront campsites on a mini-peninsula. They are well shaded, plenty far from one another, and are ideal if you want a pull-up campsite. The next nonelectric loop has sites 16–21. These are widespread and well shaded.

The other main campground road leads to the walk-in tent sites and the balance of the pull-up nonelectric sites. Walk-in tent sites 85–89 are on a loop of their own. Each one is very close to the water, offering first-rate vistas and just a short walk from your car to the camp. I would stay here anytime. Sites 90–95 are on a little knob above the water and are pull-up sites. More good pull-up sites can be found along a ridgeline—sites 96–102. These are less likely to fill because they are a bit farther away from the water.

Finally, reach the walk-in tent sites, in their own large area on a peninsula. They can be found in a variety of sites and situations. Some are directly on the water, while others are a bit back in the woods. No car-to-site walk is far, however. It can be hard to pick a site when you get here. If you want to be on the point of the peninsula, go for sites 123–127. Sites 128–131 are also lakefront.

My advice is to comb the campground for your favorite. In fact, fill your tank before you come because you are going to drive all over the place in this campground trying to

:: Ratings

BEAUTY: ★ ★ ★ ★
PRIVACY: ★ ★ ★ ★
SPACIOUSNESS: ★ ★ ★ ★
QUIET: ★ ★ ★
SECURITY: ★ ★ ★ ★ ★
CLEANLINESS: ★ ★ ★ ★

:: Key Information

ADDRESS: 954 Abbottsford Rd., LaGrange, GA 30240

OPERATED BY: U.S. Army Corps of Engineers

CONTACT: 706-884-6818, **www.sam .usace.army.mil/Missions/CivilWorks /Recreation/WestPointLake;**

RESERVATIONS: 877-444-6777, **reserveusa.com**

OPEN: Late March through early September

SITES: 35 walk-in, 16 nonelectric, 92 others

SITE AMENITIES: Picnic table, fire grate, tent pad, lantern post

ASSIGNMENT: First come, first served and by reservation

REGISTRATION: At campground entrance station

FACILITIES: Hot showers, flush toilets, water spigots

PARKING: At campsites and walk-in parking area

FEE: $16 walk-in, $24 others

ELEVATION: 650 feet

RESTRICTIONS
- **Pets:** On leash only
- **Fires:** In fire rings only
- **Alcohol:** At campsites only
- **Vehicles:** Keep cars on parking spur
- **Other:** 14-day stay limit in a 30-day period

find the absolute best site. Or reserve a site ahead of time, and then try to switch if you see something better (some campground managers hate that). All but two walk-in tent sites are reservable. After coming here once, you will find a favorite. During my trip, campers were entering the campground office and calling out for a specific site.

The campground will fill on summer holiday weekends, and, even then, the walk-in sites are the last to fill. Showers, water spigots, play areas, and restrooms are well distributed throughout the large campground. Folks from every walk of life can be found here, from families to couples to seniors. The care taken to maintain Holiday keeps them coming back.

Recreation is focused on the lake. Two boat ramps are available for camper use. In early spring, hard-core anglers enjoy Holiday. Then, everybody comes out when the weather warms, fishing for bass, bream, and crappie. Others will be out trying to beat the heat. No formal swimming area exists, but most campers swim just offshore from their campsite. Boaters will not only be fishing but waterskiing, tubing, and getting wet just about every way they can.

For land-based action, the campground has a basketball court and a tennis court. The maze of level campground roads makes for an ideal bicycling area. I like to pedal around and check out everyone's campsite setup, smell the campfires and people-watch, seeing my fellow campers enjoying life. A hiking trail runs through the campground, but I couldn't figure out exactly where it went, as it crisscrosses roads and winds around here and there. Try to figure it out for yourself. One thing you won't have to figure out, though, is that Holiday Campground is great for tent campers.

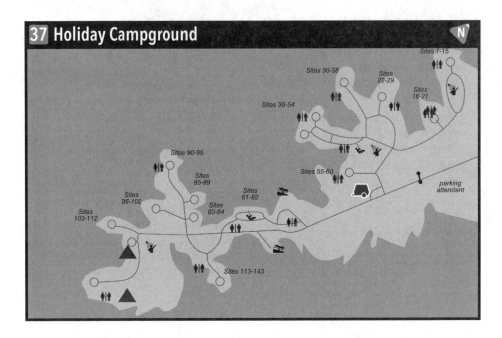

37 Holiday Campground

:: Getting There

From Exit 18 on I-85, take GA 109 West to the fountain in the square at downtown LaGrange. From there, take GA 109 West 8.7 miles to Thompson Road. Turn left on Thompson Road and follow it 0.6 mile to Abbotsford Road. Turn left on Abbottsford Road and follow it 1.6 miles to dead-end into the campground.

GPS COORDINATES   N32° 59' 55.68"   W85° 11' 37.39"

Lake Sinclair Beach Campground

This is the only Forest Service campground on Lake Sinclair.

If **Lake Sinclair Beach** were private land, it would go for big bucks. The demand for waterfront housing on the lakes outside of greater Atlanta has made that second home a pipe dream for many. There is a solution—if you have a tent. Come and enjoy Lake Sinclair at this fine Forest Service campground that is much, much cheaper than buying a lakefront lot. Located on the Little River Arm of the lake, this campground has popular waterfront sites and also some sites that allow easy water access but still offer woodsy solitude. Once here, you can enjoy the beach, relax in the sun, swim, take your boat out on the lake, or do a little hiking from the campground.

The campground is laid out in five small loops, creating a smaller, "mini-campground" atmosphere beneath the thick forest. Pass the campground entrance station and come to Loop A, with sites 1–5. It is the only loop with electricity and thus is the realm of the RV. Do be apprised that this is the Twin Bridges Trailhead (you may want to hike this path later). Next, reach Loop B, with sites 6–15. Younger hardwoods mix

with pine here, and the heavy brush and site separation allow for much privacy. Many sites require a brief walk to the camping area from the car. The loop dips to watery sites on a small creek arm of the lake. A narrow dock is available for fishing or parking your boat.

Loop C, with sites 16–26, is on the left side of the road, away from Lake Sinclair. This seems to be the forgotten loop. The sites here are the least used and offer the most solitude. Site 25 is a solitude lover's dream site.

Loop D, with sites 27–44, is the most popular loop. It has many waterfront sites overlooking the main body of the lake. Some sites here require a short walk to the camping area. The last part of the loop curves away from the lake and offers double campsites. These sites are shady but not on the water.

Bathhouses and water spigots are distributed throughout the campground. Lake Sinclair Beach fills only on summer holiday weekends. Other than that, you should be able to get a site. But first come, first served means taking your chances, so get here as early as you can on nice weather weekends. You will also get a better site if you come early. A campground host is on duty at all times.

Lake Sinclair was filled more than five decades ago. Over 417 miles of shoreline encircle 15,330 water acres. It seems to get less fishing and recreation pressure than its sister lake to the north, Lake Oconee. The Oconee River and Little River are Lake Sinclair's primary feeder branches.

:: Ratings

BEAUTY: ★ ★ ★ ★
PRIVACY: ★ ★ ★ ★
SPACIOUSNESS: ★ ★ ★
QUIET: ★ ★ ★
SECURITY: ★ ★ ★ ★
CLEANLINESS: ★ ★ ★ ★

:: Key Information

ADDRESS: Oconee Ranger District Office, 1199 Madison Rd., Eatonton, GA 31024

OPERATED BY: U.S. Forest Service

CONTACT: 706-485-1776, **www.fs.usda.gov/conf;** reservations **reserveamerica.com**

OPEN: April–November

SITES: 38 nonelectric, 6 electric

SITE AMENITIES: Picnic table, fire grate, tent pad; some have upright grills.

ASSIGNMENT: First come, first served or by reservation

REGISTRATION: At entrance station

FACILITIES: Hot showers, flush toilets, water spigots

PARKING: At campsites only

FEE: $9 nonelectric, $15 electric

ELEVATION: 365 feet

RESTRICTIONS
- **Pets:** On leash only
- **Fires:** In fire rings only
- **Alcohol:** At campsites only
- **Vehicles:** 2 vehicles per site
- **Other:** 14-day stay limit

The campground boat launch is conveniently close for all campers, and two courtesy docks aid in preparing to get on the water. The swim beach is on the point of land closest to the main body of the lake and offers the best vistas, where a changing station is conveniently located. Buoys delineate the swim area, and tan sands lead from the shoreline into the lake. A play area and picnic area are located near the beach.

Hikers can enjoy the Twin Bridges Trail, Trail 119, which leaves from Loop A. It winds through low ridges and valleys on the shoreline of Lake Sinclair. Cross a couple of bridges near the campground, and expect to pass more small creeks. There are 20 trailside interpretive stations along the way. Some gullies that the trail crosses are remnants of poor subsistence farming in the past. Other areas slice through canebrakes. Birders may find many species along the trail, which ends after 1.8 miles at a primitive camping area. Backtrack to Lake Sinclair Beach, all the while appreciating the incredible value of your inexpensive lakeside "investment."

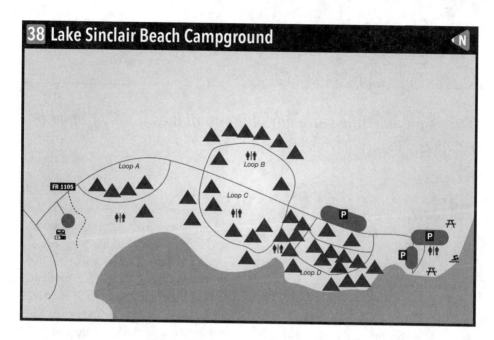

:: Getting There

From the Eatonton town square, take US 129 South 12 miles to GA 212. Turn left on GA 212 and follow it 1 mile to Twin Bridges Road. Turn left on Twin Bridges Road and follow it 1 mile to reach the campground entrance, on the left.

GPS COORDINATES   N33° 12' 22.33"   W83° 23' 57.56"

39

Magnolia Springs State Park Campground

This is an old-time state park that combines family fun with Civil War history.

Here's the recipe for a good old-fashioned family park: Start with an attractive natural setting, say a clear spring emitting millions of gallons of water daily around which grows a rich forest with wildlife aplenty, including alligators, deer, and wood storks. Overlay the land with trails from which to explore this beautiful setting. Add a lake for boating and fishing. Throw in an aquarium to view what lives underwater, and, while you're at it, install a fish hatchery nearby. Don't forget a pool for summertime swimming. Top it off with a spacious campground having just enough sites, including a few exclusively for tent campers. Finally, sprinkle in Georgia Civil War history, and you have Magnolia Springs State Park.

The campground here is appealing. It once had more than 50 sites, but that number was cut in half and each remaining site improved. Landscaping timbers delineate and level the sites, which are extra-large and extra-spacious and well separated from one another. New "fixtures" such as picnic tables,

:: Ratings

BEAUTY: ★ ★ ★
PRIVACY: ★ ★ ★
SPACIOUSNESS: ★ ★ ★ ★ ★
QUIET: ★ ★ ★
SECURITY: ★ ★ ★ ★ ★
CLEANLINESS: ★ ★ ★ ★

lantern posts, and the like were added. Tall pines tower overhead. They are spaced a bit apart, making for partial shade at some sites. Much of the ground is sand, grass, or pine needles. Occasional laurel oaks and dogwoods complement the pines. Additional shade can be had at some of the campsites that back against the dense woods surrounding most of the campground. As is often the case, the best sites are on the outside of the loop. Most of the sites are pull-in instead of pull-through.

Tent campers need to take special note of the three "walk-in" campsites that are actually drivable. They are located in thick woods on a separate narrow road of their own and have all the amenities the regular campground has, minus the electricity. The sites back there are very private and offer the best in tent camping at this park.

The main campground is also good for tent camping. The loop is centered around a bathhouse, small play area, and a screen shelter for rainy days. The screen shelter also has a stove you can use to prepare recipes of your own. A small crossroad bisects part of the inner loop and has the least appealing sites. Four sites, 13–16, back up to the park lake, which can be a mixed blessing when the motor boaters are tooling around the water on summer afternoons.

The campground fills the first Saturday in April during the Arts & Crafts/Living

:: Key Information

ADDRESS: 1053 Magnolia Springs Dr., Millen, GA 30442

OPERATED BY: Georgia State Parks

CONTACT: 478-982-1660, **gastateparks .org;** reservations 800-864-7275, **reserveamerica.com**

OPEN: Year-round

SITES: 3 walk-in, 26 others

SITE AMENITIES: Picnic table, fire ring, lantern post, tent pad, water; others also have electricity.

ASSIGNMENT: First come, first served or by reservation

REGISTRATION: At park office

FACILITIES: Hot showers, flush toilets, laundry, stove

PARKING: At campsites only

FEE: $20 walk-in, $28 all others

ELEVATION: 210 feet

RESTRICTIONS
- **Pets:** On leash only
- **Fires:** In fire rings only
- **Alcohol:** At campsites only
- **Vehicles:** 2 vehicles per site
- **Other:** 14-day stay limit

History Event, when wares are sold and a Civil War encampment is held. It will also fill on summer holiday weekends and ideal-weather spring and fall weekends. Get reservations if you can.

Now to the fun stuff. The park lake is very near the campground. You can boat around on its 28 acres, rent a boat if you don't own your own, or just bank fish. Or fish from the park pier. The lake has stiff competition for what's the best water fun. You can check out Magnolia Springs, with its clear-blue water full of fish and more turtles than I've ever seen in one place. Or check out the Bo Ginn Aquarium. Walk inside and see the assorted native and exotic fishes that roam our waters. You will likely see alligators inside the aquarium and outside around the springs. A fish hatchery is next to the aquarium, and you can walk around it to see fish being raised to feed the predatory fish of the aquarium, and others being raised for streams and lakes. Swimming is not allowed at any of the above. However, you can take a dip in the park pool, located next to the office.

Land-based recreation centers around trails that explore the land and its history. Mountain bikers will want to tackle the 5-plus-mile Hike/Bike Trail that roams the park and connects with the Beaver Trail, more popular with walkers who cruise along the lakeshore. The Woodpecker Nature Trail is near Magnolia Springs. The most interesting trail of all is the Fort Lawton Historic Trail.

The very park where we now pitch our tents and have innocent fun was a Civil War prison camp housing more than 10,000 Federal troops during a five-month period in 1864. The site was chosen due to the abundant fresh spring water and proximity to a rail line that allowed easy prisoner transport from the overcrowded, water-short, and infamous Andersonville prison. You can still see the earthworks of the fort; also check out interpretive information that gives sobering insight into our country's history. The fort tour makes us appreciate all the more what an enjoyable old-fashioned state park we have here in middle Georgia.

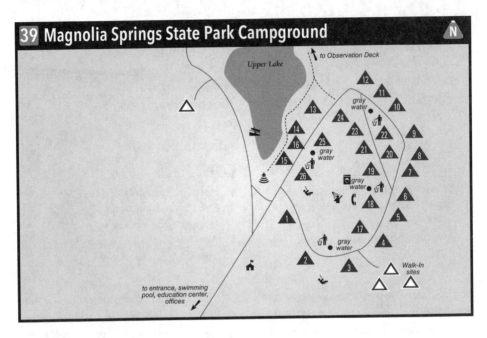

:: Getting There

From Millen, head north on US 25 5 miles to reach the park.

GPS COORDINATES   N32° 52' 58.92"   W81° 57' 10.06"

40

Oconee River Campground

This small campground offers canoeing and hiking in a rustic atmosphere.

This small Forest Service campground, which has undergone a makeover, is located along the banks of the Oconee River a few miles north of Lake Oconee. And the difference is striking. Lake Oconee can become a summertime madhouse of powerboats. The Oconee River is much quieter, receiving generally moderate use during the warm season from both self-propelled paddlers and anglers in smaller fishing boats.

The campground reflects its users—it is on the small side, quiet, and without hordes of lake lovers. Follow a spur road off GA 15 and dip into sloping land and a small flat along the Oconee River. The area is located on the outside of a bend in the river and offers a sweep both upstream and downstream. The five campsites are laid out in a small, hilly paved loop beneath a rich mixed hardwood forest of hickory, oak, dogwood, maple, and some pines. Beech and other trees form a dense understory.

Site 1 is on the inside of the small loop. Site 2 is on the outside of the loop and is on a slope. It has been leveled with landscaping timbers. Pea gravel aids in site drainage. Site 3 is inside the loop and has ample vegetation for campsite privacy, as all the sites—average in size—do. Site 4 is set back from the paved loop road. Site 5 is closest to the boat launch and the most distant from other campsites. All sites are pull-in. A vault toilet serves the campground. Bring your own water.

The boat launch and parking area are just below the campground. Bank fishermen can sometimes be seen pole in hand on a small, grassy riverside bank. A small feeder stream comes in the river here. Beech trees grow along the shoreline below the nearby picnic area, perched on a bluff overlooking the Oconee River.

Scull Shoals Trail, Trail 24, leads upstream along the right bank 1 mile to Scull Shoals Historic Area. The trail remains in the river floodplain its entire length. Here are the remains of old buildings. This settlement, begun in 1784, takes you back in time, as it was the site of Georgia's first paper mill. From here, keep north on FR 1231 and FR 1231A to pick up the Indian Mound Trail and go even farther back in time, as well as farther back from the Oconee River. Reach the first mound at 0.6 mile, with the second mound a quarter-mile beyond. The Scull Shoals Historic Area can also be reached by car. An Oconee National Forest map comes in handy for touring and for canoeing the Oconee.

Paddling is almost a must on this pretty river. The Oconee River is born in Hall

:: Ratings

BEAUTY: ★ ★ ★
PRIVACY: ★ ★ ★
SPACIOUSNESS: ★ ★ ★
QUIET: ★ ★ ★
SECURITY: ★ ★ ★
CLEANLINESS: ★ ★ ★

:: Key Information

ADDRESS: Oconee Ranger District Office, 1199 Madison Rd., Eatonton, GA 31024	**REGISTRATION:** Self-registration on-site
	FACILITIES: Vault toilet
OPERATED BY: U.S. Forest Service	**PARKING:** At campsites only
CONTACT: 706-485-1776, www.fs.usda.gov/conf	**FEE:** $5
	ELEVATION: 450 feet
OPEN: Year-round	**RESTRICTIONS**
SITES: 5	■ **Pets:** On leash only
SITE AMENITIES: Picnic table, fire grate, tent pad, lantern post	■ **Fires:** In fire rings only
	■ **Alcohol:** At campsites only
	■ **Vehicles:** 2 vehicles per site
ASSIGNMENT: First come, first served	■ **Other:** 14-day stay limit

County, then gathers strength and volume after the North and Middle Forks join it south of Athens. It then heads south for the Piedmont, flowing amid tree-lined banks. Upon entering the Oconee National Forest, the limited streamside civilization diminishes further, especially below the confluence with Big Creek. The current is generally steady and paddling is class I+. Occasional dams slow the current. Long, straight sections and gentle curves are broken by sharp bends. River width ranges between 70 and 100 feet. Heavy rains can compromise water clarity at times.

Two major paddling runs can be made on the Oconee from the campground. The upper run starts on Barnett Shoals Road at the Clarke–Oconee County line. Head downstream, passing around the Barnett Shoals Dam. Reach Oconee River Campground after 12 miles. The second run, 6.5 miles, starts at Oconee River Campground and ends at Dyar Pasture, a day-use area with a boat ramp on upper Lake Oconee below the river's confluence with Fishing Creek. The last part of the run is on slack water. Dyar Pasture has a waterfowl conservation area accessible by a 0.25-mile interpretive trail leading from the boat ramp parking area, yet another appealing locale in the Oconee National Forest.

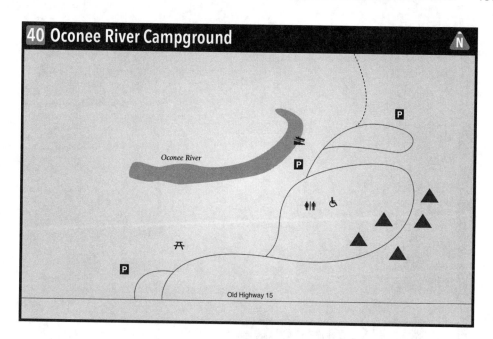

:: Getting There

From Exit 130 on I-20, take GA 44 East 2.5 miles to downtown Greensboro. Turn left on GA 15 North and follow it 12 miles to the campground, on the right. If you pass over the Oconee River Bridge, you've gone too far.

GPS COORDINATES   N33° 43' 15.07"   W83° 17' 30.54"

South
Georgia

41

Coheelee Creek Campground

This little-used southwest Georgia site is near the southernmost covered bridge in the United States.

Coheelee Creek is a seemingly forgotten backwater in southwest Georgia, flowing into the Chattahoochee River near the hamlet of Hilton. The Chattahoochee, Georgia's most significant river, is dammed as Lake George F. Andrews at this point, and forms the state border with Alabama. But looking out from Coheelee Creek Campground, you'd never know that the 'Hooch is a lake at this juncture and George W. Andrews Lock and Dam is just a few miles away. Here it is still a relatively narrow river, yet a look at the campground boat ramp reveals a small embayment backing up a short portion of Coheelee Creek, confirming the presence of a dam downstream. River or lake notwithstanding, Coheelee Creek Campground offers a quiet and quaint getaway near the most southerly covered bridge in the United States, which is 1 of only 15 original covered bridges still standing in the Peach State, and the only covered bridge south of Macon.

Pass the covered bridge before entering the campground (more about the covered bridge later). Dip through a rich forest shading Coheelee Creek to reach the boat ramp parking area. A road spurs off the parking area to reach 18 riverside campsites. The first few sites are separated from the parking area by a lush lawn. The land ends on a steep 30-foot bluff over the river. Alabama lies across the Chattahoochee. Most of the bluff is heavily vegetated, and the picnic tables are shaded. Most of the sites are directly riverside, but a low fence keeps campers from falling off the bluff. Tall laurel oaks draped in Spanish moss shade the campsites. Sweet gum and holly trees add to the tree cover. The sites themselves are average in size and a little close together, but the lack of use keeps campers adequately spaced apart.

More shaded sites are stretched along the river. None of these sites have auto pull-ins. Three parking areas are spread along the parklike camp. Campers walk a short distance to reach their sites.

A second camping area is set away from the Chattahoochee River in a deep forest of pine, laurel, oak, and magnolia. These 10 sites have auto pull-ins and are literally cut into the woods. Heavy vegetation makes for very private sites. Some of the sites only have auto pull-ins and are designed for self-contained rigs. More sites have a picnic table and lantern post. The most popular sites back here are those that spoke outward from an auto turnaround. Spring and fall are the

:: Ratings

BEAUTY: ★ ★ ★
PRIVACY: ★ ★ ★
SPACIOUSNESS: ★ ★ ★
QUIET: ★ ★ ★ ★ ★
SECURITY: ★ ★ ★
CLEANLINESS: ★ ★ ★

:: Key Information

ADDRESS: 769 Jessie Johnson St., Blakely, GA 39823	**FACILITIES:** None
OPERATED BY: Early County	**PARKING:** At campsites only
CONTACT: 229-723-4238	**FEE:** None
OPEN: Year-round	**ELEVATION:** 150 feet
SITES: 28	**RESTRICTIONS**
SITE AMENITIES: Picnic table, lantern post	■ **Pets:** On leash only
	■ **Fires:** In fire rings only
ASSIGNMENT: First come, first served	■ **Alcohol:** At campsites only
	■ **Vehicles:** 2 vehicles per site
REGISTRATION: No registration	■ **Other:** 14-day stay limit

best times to visit this park, as the gnats and mosquitoes can be troublesome in summer.

You must visit the Coheelee Creek covered bridge, which you passed on the way in. The bridge was part of the once-important Old River Road. Commissioned in 1891 at a cost of $490, this bridge eliminated the old McDonalds Ford at Coheelee Creek. The bridge fell into disrepair after the Old River Road became less used. The Daughters of the American Revolution came to the rescue and, with the help of a land donation from John Williams, established a park—Askew Park—around the bridge and the attractive cascades of Coheelee Creek. Not much else happened, until the bridge was placed on the National Register of Historic Places and restoration was completed in 1984. Askew Park, about a half-mile from the campground, certainly adds a scenic touch to the area. At the

time of my visit, some less-appreciative vandals had spray-painted part of the bridge.

Water is the center of recreation at Coheelee Creek. Local fishermen vie for crappie in the spring. Bream and bluegill are sought after in summer. Bass are present but not as plentiful as in other places. Be apprised that a current is present in the Chattahoochee River when the Army Corps of Engineers are generating at the George W. Andrews Lock and Dam downstream. Most of the time, the current is slack or imperceptible.

If you are interested in hiking trails or more history, Kolomoki Mounds State Park is half an hour away near Blakely. For more information, see the narrative for Kolomoki Mounds in this book. Then you can return to your free blufftop campsite here in Early County.

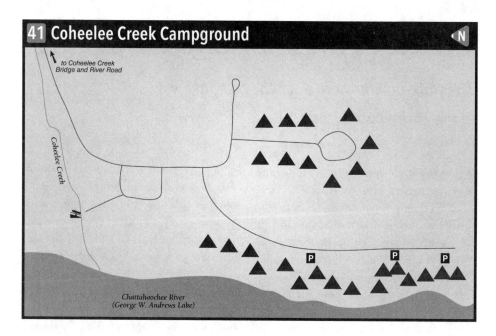

41 Coheelee Creek Campground

to Coheelee Creek
Bridge and River Road

Coheelee Creek

Chattahoochee River
(George W. Andrews Lake)

:: Getting There

From the Early County Courthouse in downtown Blakely, take GA 62 West, toward
Hilton, 10 miles to CR 25. Turn right on CR 25, and cross the railroad track, heading
forward 0.4 mile. Turn right on Old River Road, CR 278. Follow Old River Road 1
mile to the park, on your left.

GPS COORDINATES   N31° 18' 26.72"   W85° 05' 7.98"

42

Cotton Hill Campground

The walk-in sites here offer the best lake views in the entire campground.

In many instances, the U.S. Army Corps of Engineers spares no expense in constructing their campgrounds. This was evident, even though I arrived at Cotton Hill just as dusk was falling on the first warm spring evening of the year. Warm and gentle breezes were drifting off Walter F. George Lake (also referred to as Lake Eufaula) as I set up my tent at campsite 103. This site offers first-rate views of the lake, but what captured my attention were the thousands of stars emerging from the darkening sky overhead. It was simply a great time to be alive and tent camping in Georgia.

Site 103, like the others here, was chock-full of amenities—a level tent pad encircled by landscaping timbers and a cook table and grill, in addition to the standard picnic table, fire ring, and lantern post. I whipped up some burgers using the cook table, tossed them on the hot grill, and feasted during my first outdoor cookout of the year.

Site 103 is one of ten walk-in tent sites at this widespread campground, where nearly every site offers a lake view and a feeling of

solitude. The standard sites draw their share of the big rigs. Even so, there are many desirable sites other than the tent-camping sites. The whole recreation area is well manicured and meticulously maintained. Old Mill Road has 50 water and electric campsites strung along the Sandy Creek embayment. Boaters like to camp along the embayment—they can pull their watercraft directly to the shoreline without worrying about big waves off the main lake. Most sites are large and decently shaded by pines and oaks. The sites along the upper embayment are separated from the water by a field, which can be an amenity if you want to play outdoor games. Watch out for gators where the lake meets Sandy Creek. Recommended sites that can be reserved include 6, 11, 34, and 43. Sites 43–50 are good for those who want to avoid motor noise on the lake. Avoid sites 22 and 23, as they are surrounded by pavement.

Marina View, with sites 51–71, is the weakest area. Named for the George T. Bagby State Park marina it overlooks, this loop offers too many open sites and too many sites not directly lakeside, which is what you want here at Cotton Hill.

Pine Island is the place to be. This camping area, with 32 sites, looks out onto an island of pine in the lake. Nearly every campsite is directly lakeside. Tall pines shade grass and pine needles below. A sandy beach borders the lake in most places. An official swim area with buoys and the

:: Ratings

BEAUTY: ★ ★ ★ ★
PRIVACY: ★ ★
SPACIOUSNESS: ★ ★ ★ ★
QUIET: ★ ★
SECURITY: ★ ★ ★ ★ ★
CLEANLINESS: ★ ★ ★ ★

:: Key Information

ADDRESS: Route 1, Box 176, Fort Gaines, GA 31751

OPERATED BY: U.S. Army Corps of Engineers

CONTACT: 229-768-2516, **www.sam .usace.army.mil/Missions/CivilWorks /Recreation/WalterFGeorgeLakeLake GeorgeWAndrews;** reservations 877-444-6777, **reserveamerica.com**

OPEN: Year-round

SITES: 10 walk-in, 94 others

SITE AMENITIES: Picnic table, fire ring, grill, cook table, lantern post, electricity

ASSIGNMENT: First come, first served or by reservation

REGISTRATION: At gatehouse

FACILITIES: Hot showers, flush toilets, water spigots, laundry

PARKING: At walk-in parking area and campsites only

FEE: $22 walk-in, $26 others

ELEVATION: 210 feet

RESTRICTIONS

■ **Pets:** On leash only
■ **Fires:** In fire rings only
■ **Alcohol:** At campsites only
■ **Vehicles:** 3 vehicles per site
■ **Other:** 14-day stay limit

primary beach is in the center of the area and also has a playground for kids.

All the tent sites are desirable. Though lacking a little in the privacy department, the sites are spacious and offer good views. Site 104 is at the end of the campground and has good shade. Site 103 has the best views, though site 102 is nearly as good. Site 101 has a great lake view too. Shade is limited at site 100, but it is close to the swim beach. Site 99 is a sand-kick away from the beach, which would be a treat if you have kids; otherwise, it could get a little noisy during busy times. Site 98 would be good during hot times, as it is heavily shaded. Site 97 is closer to the road. Site 96 is also close to the beach. Site 95 is the last walk-in tent site. The bathrooms are a bit far from the tent area and are the only drawback for these walk-in sites. Other good sites here are located at Pine Island. The best

alternative site is 72, which has great views and is bordered by thick woods.

This is a spring, summer, and fall destination, though winter is best for quiet. It can fill on spring break. Fishing is the main attraction here on Walter F. George Lake. Crappie, catfish, and bass are the primary game fish. A wide boat ramp and fish-cleaning station make catching and cleaning your fish easier. The wide, level, and lightly used campground roads are excellent for the casual bicycler. Because the campground is so large, there are enough roads to keep the wheeled set plenty busy. Walking is another land pursuit. A short nature trail circles around a wetland and over a boardwalk before completing its loop. The swim beach is a big draw during summer. No matter what time of year you visit, something draws you to Cotton Hill.

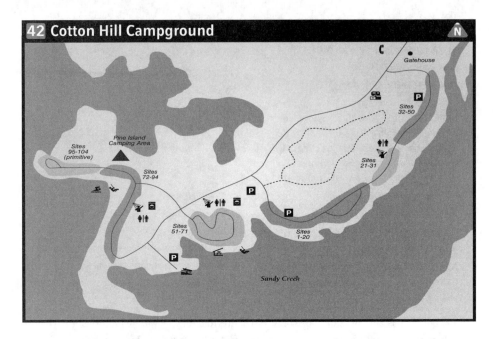

:: Getting There

From the intersection of GA 37 and GA 39 in Fort Gaines, take GA 39 North 9 miles to a signed left turn. Turn left and travel just a short distance, taking your next left to enter the campground after 0.7 mile.

GPS COORDINATES N31° 40' 25.83"   W85° 03' 49.47"

43

Fort McAllister State Historic Park Campground

Camp on a coastal barrier island at the end of a dead-end road.

Everybody's **heard** of Sherman's March to the Sea, the Union movement across Georgia during the Civil War. This march ended the Confederates' quest for a country of their own. The march stopped here at Fort McAllister, the final battleground before Sherman headed into Savannah. Later, Henry Ford bought the land and preserved Fort McAllister. Next, a timber company bought the land from Ford's estate and donated the fort to the state of Georgia. Today, we have not only a state-run historic site that allows insight into coastal defenses of the War Between the States but also a fine campground with a tent-only area on a small barrier island at the end of a dead-end road.

In the early days of the war, none other than Robert E. Lee, head Confederate honcho, inspected Fort McAllister, on the lower Ogeechee River, and offered ideas to beef up its defenses. His ideas proved worthwhile, as the fort stayed in Rebel hands until Sherman's fateful march, despite several attacks from Federal gunboats, including

the new-for-the-time ironclads. And if it weren't for the fort, this area would probably not have been preserved. So tour the fort with multiple layers of appreciation.

The campground itself is a big draw— I loved it. It is located on Savage Island, attached to the mainland by a causeway traversing the salt marsh and creeks that encircle the island. This makes for a peaceful and serene camping experience. A hiking trail and boat ramp offer immediate recreation, whereas other park offerings, including the fort, are located on the mainland. Thus, Savage Island acts as an oasis for the campers.

The campground is laid out in a grand loop cut by crossroads. The first area has 18 sites that are RV-land. The helpful campground host stays here. However, you can appreciate the setting that defines the island: live oaks, stately magnolias, laurel oaks, palms, and pines draped in Spanish moss. Far-reaching salt marshes broken by tidal creeks surround Savage Island. Ample understory vegetation enhances campsite privacy among these very large campsites that are all pull-through. The first crossroad, Raccoon Way, has sites 19–38. It is well shaded but caters to the big rigs. The better crossroad is Armadillo Avenue, which houses sites 39–52. The sites here are extremely large. The tent camper's area is at the farthest end of the island on Deer Run. I stayed in campsite 53, as it was closest to the

:: Ratings

BEAUTY: ★ ★ ★ ★
PRIVACY: ★ ★ ★
SPACIOUSNESS: ★ ★ ★ ★
QUIET: ★ ★ ★ ★
SECURITY: ★ ★ ★ ★ ★
CLEANLINESS: ★ ★ ★

:: Key Information

ADDRESS: 3894 Fort McAllister Rd., Richmond Hill, GA 31324

OPERATED BY: Georgia State Parks

CONTACT: 912-727-2339, **gastateparks .org;** reservations 800-864-7275, **reserveamerica.com**

OPEN: Year-round

SITES: 12 tent-only, 52 others

SITE AMENITIES: Picnic table, fire grate, tent pad, water, electricity

ASSIGNMENT: First come, first served or by reservation

REGISTRATION: At park office

FACILITIES: Hot showers, flush toilets, laundry, phone

PARKING: At campsites only

FEE: $27 tent, $30 others

ELEVATION: 7 feet

RESTRICTIONS
- **Pets:** On leash only
- **Fires:** In fire rings only
- **Alcohol:** At campsites only
- **Vehicles:** 2 vehicles per site
- **Other:** 14-day stay limit

water, which is still a good walk away. Continue down the row and the sites become more heavily shaded. Tent pads keep the water from ponding under you during a storm. Of special note is campsite 63. It is the largest site and offers the most privacy.

Reservations are recommended on all holiday weekends from St. Patrick's Day through Thanksgiving. Campsites are generally otherwise available at this serene, marsh-encircled setting, where the birds will wake you instead of an alarm clock.

Recreation is immediate from your tent site on Savage Island. The Magnolia Nature Trail starts near the end of the tent area and loops around to return to the campground. If you've ever wanted to try sea kayaking, here's your chance. The park rents kayaks and canoes at very reasonable rates. Explore the marsh creeks, starting from the boat landing on Red Bird Creek. Try to work the tides in your favor. Kayaking is deservedly catching on in these parts, and the launch is open to bigger boats too. Bicycles can also be rented inexpensively. The flat and quiet park roads make for fun pedaling, especially on the causeway overlooking the expansive

marshes. Registered campers can fish from the dock/boat ramp near the campground.

The Red Bird Trail system is back on the mainland. The system offers a series of interconnected loops that traverse the rich forest and marshland protected by the park. It is open to hikers and bikers. A 90-foot fishing pier is located on the Ogeechee River. Here, you can go for whiting, sea trout, drum, and even sharks. Crabbers also try their luck here.

You simply can't miss touring Fort McAllister and the adjacent museum located in the park office. The views from the fort are inspiring. Learn about a soldier's life at this once-lonely outpost, broken by sporadic gun battles with the Union. Consider how the soldiers used the material on hand for what were then state-of-the-art fortifications. Check out the gun emplacements and massive earthworks and underground quarters called "bombproofs." The Overseer's House is next to the fort. How times have changed. Luckily for us, this preserve is one place where we can pitch our tent, relax on a barrier island, and consider days gone by, among other things.

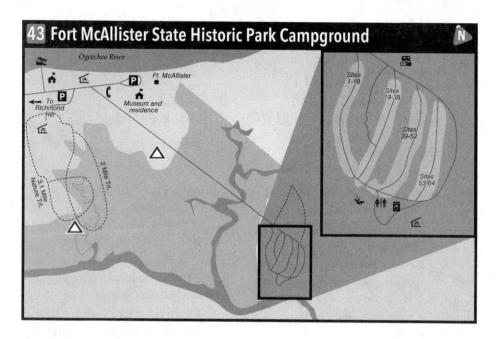

:: Getting There

From Exit 90 on I-95, take GA 144 East 6.6 miles, to the GA 144 Spur. Turn left on the GA 144 Spur and follow it 4 miles to dead-end at the state park.

GPS COORDINATES   N31° 53' 24.11"   W81° 11' 52.70"

44

General Coffee State Park Campground

This unheralded Georgia state park combines natural beauty with a living-history farm.

The folks down in Coffee County are quite proud of their area, and deservedly so. They banded together in the 1960s to preserve and donate a portion of their domain to establish General Coffee State Park, named after their native son, John Coffee (who was an area settler in the early 1800s, state legislature member, and later a U.S. Congressman who earned his generalship fighting Native Americans), for whom the county is also named. Located in the sandhills and swamp forest ecosystem along the Seventeen Mile River, this park has a fine campground to complement its natural features and an on-site living-history farm. This park is not only about places but also about people. General Coffee State Park has many local and repeat visitors, so much so that the friendly park staff knows many of them on a first-name basis. I was welcomed as a friend and enjoyed my stay at this quiet and underutilized venue, where campers explore the park trails, waters, and log structures of the Heritage Farm.

:: Ratings

BEAUTY: ★ ★ ★
PRIVACY: ★ ★
SPACIOUSNESS: ★ ★
QUIET: ★ ★ ★ ★
SECURITY: ★ ★ ★ ★ ★
CLEANLINESS: ★ ★ ★ ★

Before you explore this Georgia gem, first pitch your tent. The 50-site campground is divided into two loops in a forest of young laurel oaks, turkey oaks, and pine trees. Spanish moss drapes from the tree limbs. The understory is limited to some palmetto, but the abundance of trees and lack of heavy use make campsite privacy less of an issue. A bathhouse, grass lawn, and small playground centers each loop. Generally, the sites on the outside of the loop are most desirable, as they face the attractive woods. All sites are pull-through. Campground hosts and on-site rangers provide good security.

Surprisingly, the campground only fills on summer holiday weekends. You can get a site just about any other weekend and expect to not have any next-door neighbors. According to the park manager, the best months to visit are April, May, October, and November.

I stayed in campsite 39 because it was close to the Gopher Loop, one of the two primary trails here. This path travels through a part of the park that protects the gopher tortoise and indigo snake, which like the sand hills environment. The other trail, the River Trail, connects the campground with the rest of the park. Here, you cruise along the meshing zone of the sandhills and the swamp forest and along the Seventeen Mile River. This watercourse is a swamp river and can be seen close-up from

:: Key Information

ADDRESS: 46 John Coffee Rd., Nicholls, GA 51554

OPERATED BY: Georgia State Parks

CONTACT: 912-384-7082, **gastateparks .org;** reservations 800-864-7275, **reserveamerica.com**

OPEN: Year-round

SITES: 50

SITE AMENITIES: Picnic table, fire grate, water, electricity; some also have grills.

ASSIGNMENT: First come, first served or by reservation

REGISTRATION: At park office

FACILITIES: Hot showers, flush toilets, laundry, phone

PARKING: At campsites only

FEE: $26

ELEVATION: 230 feet

RESTRICTIONS
- **Pets:** On leash only
- **Fires:** In fire rings only
- **Alcohol:** At campsites only
- **Vehicles:** 2 vehicles per site
- **Other:** 6 persons per campsite

the boardwalk, which crosses the river near picnic shelter 5. The river was up during my stay and the dark waters flowed strongly below the boardwalk.

The Heritage Farm not only contains original log structures but also live animals and smaller outbuildings where you can see how things were done in General Coffee's day. Check out the smokehouse, the cane mill, the blacksmith shop, and the turpentine-making station. Tools and other items of those days complement the buildings. The Meeks Cabin was built in 1828 and is reputed to be the oldest standing log structure in south Georgia. The full-time park naturalist can usually be found in the Relihan Cabin, which mixes old-time displays with natural history exhibits.

A special note: Pioneer Skills Day is held the third Saturday in October. Then,

Heritage Farm is alive with demonstrations of bygone days from the 1860s to the 1930s. Smaller-scale park programs are held nearly every weekend. The Jefferson Davis State Historic Site is about 40 miles distant, near Fitzgerald. Here is where the president of the Confederacy was captured after abandoning Richmond.

The park lake, adjacent to the Heritage Farm, offers canoeing and fishing. Boats are available for rent, as are bicycles for those who like to pedal the park roads. Bicycles are also allowed on the River Trail, but take it easy on the speed. The park swimming pool is open from Memorial Day to Labor Day, offering a respite from the hot summer days. General Coffee State Park can be your haven, and you'll understand why it's the pride of Coffee County.

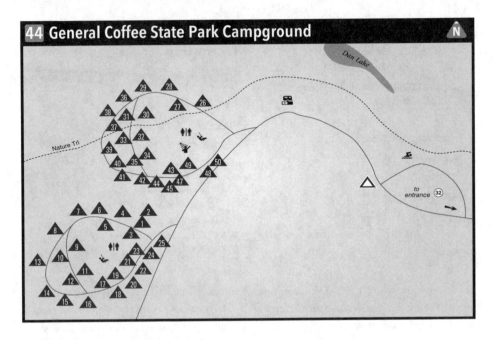

:: Getting There

From Douglas, take GA 32 East 4 miles to the state park, on your left.

GPS COORDINATES   N31° 31' 28.43"   W82° 45' 47.47"

45

Kolomoki Mounds State Historic Park Campground

This quiet, historic park is a great spring getaway, but it's also fun in the fall.

Tent campers are far from being the first ones to overnight here. American Indians had a village here at least 1,000 years ago. During their time here, these aboriginal Americans built mounds that still stand today and are the reason for this state park. After purchasing this land from the Mercier family, the state of Georgia added recreational facilities to complement the historic nature of the Kolomoki Mounds. The facilities include two campgrounds where you can pitch your tent, then explore both the human and natural history of this southwest Peach State preserve.

The park once had two campgrounds, but the higher-ups in Atlanta closed the old Tall Pines Campground, leaving us with Lake Kolomoki Campground. Lake Kolomoki is laid out in a classic loop with pull-in and pull-through campsites. Sites 1–11 are stretched directly along the water. Unfortunately, shade is limited. Site 11 is the exception and is shaded and scenic. Site 18 has shade and solitude. The loop curves away

:: Ratings

BEAUTY:	★ ★ ★
PRIVACY:	★ ★
SPACIOUSNESS:	★ ★ ★ ★
QUIET:	★ ★ ★ ★
SECURITY:	★ ★ ★
CLEANLINESS:	★ ★ ★

from the lake and climbs a small hill past a new bathhouse. The sites back here are less popular than the lakeside sites.

The campground fills on summer holiday weekends and during the Kolomoki Festival, the second weekend in October.

Your first order of business is to check out the mounds, the reason for this park's existence. You may want to explore the mound museum first. It actually sits atop an excavated mound, left as the scientists pored through it. Here you can examine the layout of what was found under the earth and explore the theories as to why and how the mounds were built. Next, take the self-guided walking tour of the mounds. Temple Mound stands far above the rest at 56 feet in height and more than 200 feet at its base. Mound D once housed a revered leader, servants, slaves, trophy skulls, and the leader's wives. Oddly enough, one mound contains members of the Mercier family. You'll have to learn the rest of that story yourself.

Recreational pastimes are plentiful at the park. Two lakes, formed by damming Kolomoki Creek, offer watery fun. You already know about Lake Kolomoki. Fishing is popular here and is made easier with park boats for rent. Check out fishing gear from the park office. Pedal boats, johnboats, and canoes can be plied along the lake in search of bass, bream, crappie, and catfish. Lake Yohola is upstream of Lake Kolomoki and

:: Key Information

ADDRESS: 205 Indian Mounds Rd., Blakely, GA 39823

OPERATED BY: Georgia State Parks

CONTACT: 229-724-2150, **gastateparks.org;** reservations 800-864-7275, **reserveamerica.com**

OPEN: Year-round

SITES: 25

SITE AMENITIES: Picnic table, fire grate, water, electricity

ASSIGNMENT: First come, first served or by reservation

REGISTRATION: At park office

FACILITIES: Hot showers, flush toilets, water spigots, laundry

PARKING: At campsites only

FEE: $28

ELEVATION: 300 feet

RESTRICTIONS

- **Pets:** On leash only
- **Fires:** In fire rings only
- **Alcohol:** At campsites only
- **Vehicles:** None
- **Other:** Park offers monthly and weekly camping rates

offers fishing too. Swimming is prohibited due to the presence of alligators. But fear not, for the park offers a large swimming pool where you can get wet without worrying about what lies beneath.

In addition to the mounds walking tour, you can also walk a 1.5-mile trail that skirts the north shore of Lake Kolomoki, or take the 3-mile Swift Creek Trail, which explores both lakes. This orange-blazed path features bird-watching platforms where you can secretly and quietly observe winged wildlife. If you are in the mood for a little competition, challenge your fellow tent campers to some miniature golf. Admittedly, miniature golf is quite a departure from the days when aboriginal Americans camped here, building the mounds that make this park special.

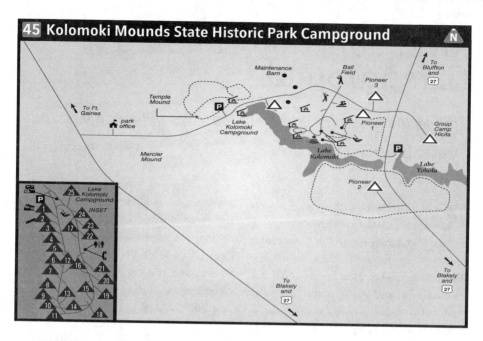

:: Getting There

From the Early County courthouse in Blakely, take US 27 Business North 2.2 miles to First Kolomoki Road. Turn left onto First Kolomoki Road, CR 280, and follow it 4.4 miles to reach the park, on your right.

GPS COORDINATES   N31° 28' 3.92"   W84° 55' 41.61"

46

River Junction Landing Campground

This secluded locale can be your base camp for enjoying the greater Lake Seminole area.

River Junction Landing is a quiet getaway that makes for a great base camp on Lake Seminole, located in the extreme southwest corner of Georgia, where the Peach State meets Florida and Alabama. Its small size and rustic nature are more typical of a rougher area, but here the campground is patrolled by a campground host and has hot showers to boot. So pitch your tent, explore this large lake without worry, and when you come back, the fabulous hot showers will be waiting for you!

As you enter the camping area, the road splits. Six campsites are situated in the center of a rectangular loop road. Laurel oaks, water oaks, and pines shade these six sites. Understory vegetation is limited, but the lack of use at the campground makes privacy less of an issue than other places. Site 1, my choice, offers distance from other sites and proximity to the bathhouse. Site 2 is closer to the boat landing but is still on the bluff. Sites 3 and 4 are a bit close together, as

are sites 5 and 6. Sites 7–11 are poor. They are merely wide paved spots on the outside of the loop road where trailers can pull up; they have no tables, grills, or other amenities. Sites 12 and 13 do not exist. The last three campsites are set along the sloping road that drops off the bluff to the campground boat ramp. Site 14 offers the most solitude. Site 15 requires a short walk from the boat-ramp parking area. Site 16 also requires a short walk but is closest to the boat ramp.

River Junction Landing is underutilized. When I asked the campground host how often the campground fills, he shook his head and said, "Never," then went on to explain, "Stragglers just dribble in here and there."

A second camping area nearby is free. On the way in, 13 miles from Bainbridge on GA 97, you passed the right turn to Faceville Landing. This camp and day-use area is lower and closer to the water and is set on the embayment of a creek beneath pines, oaks, and magnolia trees. The six sites here are a bit rougher, and the facilities consist of a water spigot in the picnic area and a vault toilet. There are no showers and no campground host, but the landing does have a picnic shelter, which can be handy during bouts of rain. A boat ramp offers easy access to Seminole Lake.

The shoreline of this lake will surprise you. Steep bluffs border much of the

:: Ratings

BEAUTY: ★ ★ ★
PRIVACY: ★ ★
SPACIOUSNESS: ★ ★ ★ ★
QUIET: ★ ★ ★ ★
SECURITY: ★ ★ ★
CLEANLINESS: ★ ★ ★

:: Key Information

ADDRESS: P.O. Box 96, Chattahoochee, FL 32324	**REGISTRATION:** Self-registration on-site
OPERATED BY: U.S. Army Corps of Engineers	**FACILITIES:** Hot showers, flush toilets, water spigots
CONTACT: 229-662-2001, **www.sam .usace.army.mil/Missions/CivilWorks /Recreation/LakeSeminole**	**PARKING:** At campsites only
	FEE: $18
OPEN: Year-round	**ELEVATION:** 140 feet
SITES: 9 tent sites, 5 others	**RESTRICTIONS**
SITE AMENITIES: Picnic table, fire grate, grill, lantern post, trash can	■ **Pets:** On leash only ■ **Fires:** In fire rings only ■ **Alcohol:** At campsites only
ASSIGNMENT: First come, first served	■ **Vehicles:** None ■ **Other:** 14-day stay limit

shoreline. River Junction Landing Campground is located on one such bluff. The river junction referred to at this particular spot is the confluence of the Flint River and Spring Creek—both watercourses form arms of the lake.

Seminole Lake is formed by the confluence of the Chattahoochee, the primary river of Georgia, and the Flint River, plus a few smaller streams, such as Spring Creek. Together, they drain more than 17,000 square miles of land. This attractive lake has 376 miles of shoreline, and that makes for plenty of opportunities to enjoy fishing, boating, and swimming. Both Faceville Landing and River Junction Landing have boat ramps. River Junction Landing has a small courtesy dock, which is also great for looking out on the lake or lazy bank fishing.

Having a campground host on location kept me at ease while I explored other parts of the lake. Other nearby attractions on Lake Seminole include the Jim Woodruff Lock and Dam, which forms Lake Seminole. There's a nice bank-fishing area just below the dam. Chattahoochee Park, on a point overlooking the lake not far from River Junction Landing, is a day-use area with a swim beach, boat ramp, playground, and nature trail. Westbank Overlook is just on the far side of the dam. Yet more attractions lie up the Chattahoochee River arm of the lake, as well as the Flint River arm of the lake. It pays to call ahead for an Army Corps of Engineers Lake Seminole map if you want to branch out. And branching out here is easy to do from your comfy base camp at River Junction Landing.

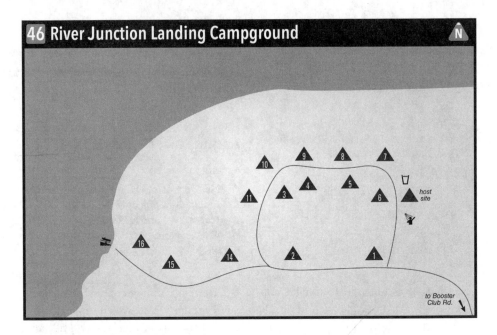

46 River Junction Landing Campground

:: Getting There

From US 27 on the western edge of Bainbridge, take GA 97, Faceville Highway, west 15 miles. Turn right on the GA 97 Spur and follow it 1.8 miles to Booster Club Road. Turn left on Booster Club Road and follow it 8 miles to River Junction Landing Road. Turn right here and follow it to dead-end into the campground.

GPS COORDINATES N30° 44' 57.60"   W84° 50' 26.53"

47

Rood Creek Campground

The campsites here are lakeside—and free!

Upon entering Rood Creek, I slowly and casually drove through the campground, looking for a site. It was a late Saturday afternoon and the campground was mostly full. Folks were sitting at picnic tables, lounging in their chairs, and rustling up dinner inside screen shelters. Campfire smoke was wafting through the trees. One fellow was standing before his group, talking animatedly. During his story he stretched out his arms. He stretched and stretched, and to my surprise, his arms were longer than his legs! Turns out that he was describing the fish that had gotten away earlier in the day. As I looked around, nearly everyone camped here had these extremely long arms, which stretched way beyond the norm. I asked myself, "How could all these people possibly have these unusually long arms?" I finally put it all together—Rood Creek is a fisherman's campground!

The above story may be a stretch, but it is no stretch that it is mostly anglers who use this free Army Corps of Engineers campground on the Rood Creek arm of Walter F. George Lake, commonly known as Lake Eufaula. Nearly all the campsites here are

:: Ratings

BEAUTY: ★ ★ ★ ★
PRIVACY: ★ ★ ★
SPACIOUSNESS: ★ ★ ★
QUIET: ★ ★ ★
SECURITY: ★ ★ ★
CLEANLINESS: ★ ★ ★

directly on a lakeside bluff 10 feet or so above the water. This arm of the lake is relatively narrow and makes the area seem more intimate than other spots overlooking a lake with 640 miles of shoreline, such as Lake Eufaula.

Enter the camping area and go forward to reach a boat ramp separating the campground. Fourteen non-numbered sites are to your right. The first eight overlook the lake and are separated from one another by vegetation. Though the lake view is nice, the view of the boat ramp parking area on the landward side of the campsites detracts a bit from these eight sites. The shoreline curves toward six more campsites. These are spaced at different distances from the lake and are often used for double campsites. The last site is the best. It is on the water, wooded on its back side, and is shaded by a big magnolia overhead.

Turn left from the boat ramp to reach the loop portion of the campground, with 20 more sites. Pines, sweet gum, laurel oak, maple, and magnolia shade the shoreline. Spanish moss sways from the tree limbs. These sites are better in general, though a few are a bit close together. The loop curves to reach some sites on a point that are highly coveted. The sites then become unevenly spaced from the lake, though all are no more than 20 feet from the water. The final area has four sites on a dead-end road. These sites are well separated from one another, yet all are lakeside. This is where I stayed, seeking privacy and quiet after a hectic time getting out of Atlanta.

:: Key Information

ADDRESS: Route 1, Box 176, Fort Gaines, GA 31751	**ASSIGNMENT:** First come, first served
OPERATED BY: U.S. Army Corps of Engineers	**REGISTRATION:** No registration
CONTACT: 912-768-2516, **www.sam .usace.army.mil/Missions/CivilWorks /Recreation/WalterFGeorgeLakeLake GeorgeWAndrews**	**FACILITIES:** Vault toilets (bring your own water)
	PARKING: At campsites only
OPEN: Year-round	**FEE:** None
SITES: 34	**ELEVATION:** 210 feet
SITE AMENITIES: Picnic table, lantern post; most also have upright grill and fire ring.	**RESTRICTIONS**
	■ **Pets:** On leash only
	■ **Fires:** In fire rings only
	■ **Alcohol:** At campsites only
	■ **Vehicles:** None
	■ **Other:** 14-day stay limit

The loop portion of the campground is closed December through February. The campground fills on weekends when the crappie are biting—mid-March through mid-April. Rood Creek will also fill on summer holiday weekends. Otherwise, you can generally get a site at this free campground.

A boat ramp is conveniently located for all campers. Though the campground is free, there is a small fee for use of the boat ramp. A courtesy dock aids entry and exit into the lake. Some campers pull their boats to their campsite and tie them to shore. The main body of Lake Eufaula is just out of sight from the camping area.

Fishing and telling fishing tales are the main activities here at Rood Creek. Families, friends, and an occasional outdoor writer up for some low-key fishing are mixed in with the hard-core anglers. Crappie are the fish of choice in spring. Largemouth bass are a big draw too. In summer, anglers of all ages will go for bream or catfish.

Providence Canyon State Conservation Park, one of Georgia's most underrated and underutilized hiking resources, is just a few minutes away. Known as the Little Grand Canyon, this unusual landscape was formed by erosive farming practices of the 1800s. This erosion cut gullies into the soil, exposing a surprising array of colors in these canyons, some as deep as 150 feet. Three miles of trails are open for hiking, as well as a 7-mile backcountry trail, a camping destination in its own right. You likely passed signs to Providence Canyon on the way to Rood Creek. To access the park from Rood Creek, head north on GA 39 to GA 39C. Turn right on GA 39C and follow it 8 miles to Providence Canyon, yet another reason to visit southwest Georgia.

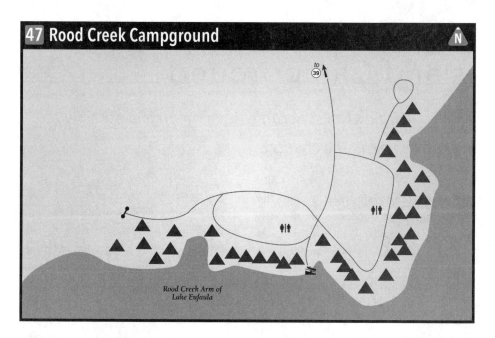

47 Rood Creek Campground

Rood Creek Arm of Lake Eufaula

:: Getting There

From the intersection of GA 27 and GA 39 in Georgetown, take GA 39 North 6.4 miles to CR 107. Turn left on CR 107 and follow it 1.4 miles to dead-end at the campground.

GPS COORDINATES   N32° 01' 30.25"   W85° 02' 11.20"

48

Sea Camp at Cumberland Island Campground

This is Georgia's finest ocean tent camping and possibly the best anywhere in the country.

Cumberland Island is a must for Georgia tent campers—out-of-staters too. This barrier island, the southernmost in the Peach State, is special. The scenery is magnificent—from the windswept beaches to the massive live oaks shading palmetto thickets to the wild horses to the historic mansions. From your base camp, you can explore Cumberland Island on foot trails aplenty, relax on the beach, or enjoy the many interpretive programs offered by the park service that delve into the deep history of this island.

The campground, Sea Camp, matches the exceptional beauty of the island. However, before you see the campground, you must go through a short ranger orientation after which you will be given your campsite. Then, you load your stuff onto carts provided by the park service to haul your gear from the landward side of the island to the seaward side of the island, a few hundred yards.

The first segment of the campground, sites 1–12, curves into a forest of live oaks

:: Ratings

BEAUTY: ★ ★ ★ ★ ★
PRIVACY: ★ ★ ★ ★ ★
SPACIOUSNESS: ★ ★ ★ ★
QUIET: ★ ★ ★ ★ ★
SECURITY: ★ ★ ★ ★ ★
CLEANLINESS: ★ ★ ★ ★ ★

behind dunes leading to the Atlantic. Massive tree trunks divide into incredibly long limbs under which grow chest-high palmetto and wax myrtle. Spanish moss hangs below the oak limbs, and ferns grow atop them. The campsites are literally cut out from the thick ground vegetation, ensuring maximum privacy. You will immediately notice the unusual elevated food storage boxes. The raccoons here are particularly adept at getting at human food, so the park service installed these boxes, which every camper must use. Most campsites are heavily shaded and more than adequate for whatever supplies you can bring on the ferry.

By the way, there are no stores on the island, and you must bring everything you need with you (you must also pack out all of your trash). Load up on ice and groceries. The campground does provide water. Spigots are spread throughout the campground. This campground segment ends near a small outdoor picnic/interpretive area where ranger programs are held. A bathhouse near the campground center has cold indoor showers and flush toilets. Outdoor showers are available near the boardwalk to the beach.

The second area has sites 13–16. All the sites here are a tad closer to the beach but are not necessarily better. They, too, are shaded by live oaks and well separated

:: Key Information

ADDRESS: P.O. Box 806, St. Mary's, GA 31558

OPERATED BY: National Park Service

CONTACT: 912-882-4336, **nps.gov/cuis;** reservations, 912-882-4335; ferry reservations, 877-860-6787 weekdays 10 a.m.–4 p.m.

OPEN: Year-round

SITES: 16

SITE AMENITIES: Picnic table, fire ring, raccoon-proof food-storage box, trash-storage pole

ASSIGNMENT: First come, first served or by reservation

REGISTRATION: At camper check-in on island

FACILITIES: Cold indoor and outdoor showers, flush toilets, water spigots

PARKING: At lot near ferry to Cumberland Island

FEE: $4 per person per night, plus $4 park entrance fee

ELEVATION: 15 feet

RESTRICTIONS
- **Pets:** Not advised, not allowed on ferry
- **Fires:** In fire rings only
- **Alcohol:** At campsites only
- **Vehicles:** None allowed on island
- **Other:** 7-day stay limit; also pack it in, pack it out

from one another. Simply put, there is not a bad campsite on this island—I would stay in any one of them. And make no mistake about it, this campground is popular. Business is steady year-round, despite the heat and bugs of summer and sporadic cold snaps of winter. The campground is likely to fill almost every weekend of the year, but this is weather-dependent. Reservations can be made six months in advance and are highly recommended. In summer, stays are generally shorter than the seven-day limit. In winter, the ferry doesn't run on Mondays or Tuesdays, altering the visitation patterns a bit. All of my visits were in spring, and I loved every one of them.

The beach is a big draw. Nearly every barrier island in the state has been or is being developed. Cumberland Island does have some private inholdings, but the vast majority of it is in nature's hands only. The beach will stack up to any other on the East Coast and is a huge draw. The interior of the island has its beauty, too, with the live oak and pine woods broken by wetter sections and inland ponds. Miles and miles of trails traverse the island from one end to the other. Wild horses roam the island, and it's exciting to see them. You may also encounter deer, wild turkeys, and slow-moving armadillos.

The River Trail leads south from the park office to the Dungeness Dock and the Dungeness Historic District. This historic area is the site of two former mansions, both with the mysterious name of Dungeness. The first one was built by Revolutionary War hero Nathanael Greene and the second by businessman Thomas Carnegie. There are more than ruins here, but you will have to explore for yourself and learn of a way of life gone by. Better yet, join a ranger for one of the twice-daily interpretive walks. On the upper end of the island are Plum Orchard, an intact mansion, and The Settlement. Park tours of Plum Orchard and The Settlement are held monthly. And after one trip here, you will definitely want to visit Cumberland Island monthly.

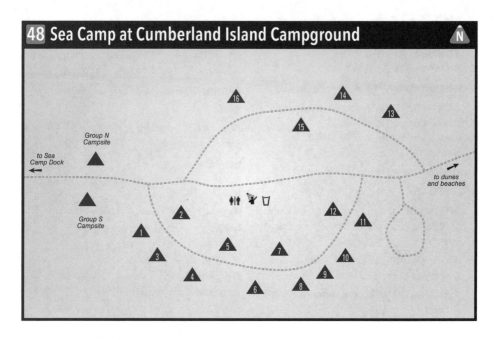

:: Getting There

From Exit 3 on I-95, take GA 40 East 10 miles to dead-end in St. Mary's near the park's visitor center and private ferry. You must then take the ferry to Cumberland Island.

GPS COORDINATES   N30° 46' 40.12"   W81° 28' 2.75"

49

Skidaway Island State Park Campground

This barrier island park offers natural beauty and quick access to historic Savannah.

You never know what you may find at a state park. Here at Skidaway Island, I was expecting a quality coastal camping experience, but I also found a 20-foot-tall ground sloth—a replica, that is—of the tallest land mammal that ever lived. See, back in the ground sloth's day, more than 10,000 years ago, these creatures roamed the coastal plain, among other places, feeding on tree vegetation. In 1823, the slaves of an area planter named Stark alerted him to some odd and large bones. Soon these bones became famous as the first giant sloth bones to be found. Now you can see a replica of this skeleton, among other interesting things, at the interpretive museum, which also focuses on wild birds, the currently featured living critters in these parts. Skidaway Island is an important stop on the Georgia Coastal Birding Trail.

Animals aside, this state park does have a fine campground on its 553 acres, which one park staffer described as a "pocket park of what used to be." Georgia's coast is growing rapidly, and Skidaway Island is no exception. Civilization is at the park's doorstep. The campground mixes a few civilized amenities into a very pretty forest of fern-covered live oaks, tall pines, and palms draped in Spanish moss. Yaupon, wax myrtle, and palmetto make for much brush between campsites. At first, I was alarmed that the park has 88 campsites, but they are widespread over a very large area, so large you may get lost driving on the winding roads among the four camping areas.

All sites are pull-through and widely separated, allowing for privacy and spaciousness. Three comfort stations are conveniently located in the campground. Sites 41–65 are of special note, offering more lush vegetation along a creek. They are also lower lying, but tent pads will keep you high and dry during the wettest times. There is no avoiding the big rigs here, as they scatter throughout the campground.

The campground will fill on holiday weekends from St. Patrick's Day through Thanksgiving. Make reservations well in advance if you are coming then. Otherwise, sites are generally available. Spring and fall are the busiest and best times to visit.

Campers like to stay here not only for the park but also for its proximity to Savannah, which has one of the largest historic

:: Ratings

BEAUTY: ★ ★ ★
PRIVACY: ★ ★ ★
SPACIOUSNESS: ★ ★ ★
QUIET: ★ ★
SECURITY: ★ ★ ★ ★ ★
CLEANLINESS: ★ ★ ★ ★

:: Key Information

ADDRESS: 52 Diamond Causeway, Savannah, GA 31411	**REGISTRATION:** At park office
OPERATED BY: Georgia State Parks	**FACILITIES:** Hot showers, flush toilets, laundry, phone
CONTACT: 912-598-2300, **gastateparks .org;** reservations 800-864-7275, **reserveamerica.com**	**PARKING:** At campsites only
	FEE: $35–$45
OPEN: Year-round	**ELEVATION:** 8 feet
SITES: 88	**RESTRICTIONS**
SITE AMENITIES: Picnic table, fire grate, tent pad, water, electricity, cable hookup	■ **Pets:** On leash only ■ **Fires:** In fire rings only ■ **Alcohol:** At campsites only
ASSIGNMENT: First come, first served or by reservation	■ **Vehicles:** 2 vehicles per site ■ **Other:** 14-day stay limit

preservation districts in the country. Colonial and Civil War history converge in this coastal town that played a critical role in Georgia's past. Speaking of history, don't miss Wormsloe, the nearby home of colonial settler Noble Jones. He arrived here in 1733, carving out a life on the Isle of Hope in what was then a howling wilderness.

Back to the sloth and the interpretive museum. Besides the sloth, the museum offers an introduction to birding. The painted bunting is an especially attractive bird that makes the rounds here. A spotting scope is trained on a feeder just outside the museum. Binoculars, bird books, and taped bird songs aid in your learning experience. Then you'll be ready to tackle some birding and historical discovery on the 5 miles of trails here. The Sandpiper Trail travels through several ecosystems, which enhances your birding opportunities. Smaller birds will be out along Avian Way,

larger shorebirds out by the Skidaway Narrows, where boats pass on the Intracoastal Waterway. Check out the Confederate Earthworks set up to defend the waterways during the Civil War. Short on defenses, Johnny Reb may have used what is known as a Quaker cannon to deter the Union. Soldiers would cut down palm trees and paint them black to make them look like cannons, providing a mirage of increased defense! An observation tower allows more visuals of the salt marsh.

The Big Ferry Interpretive Trail is longer and departs from near the campground. There's an old liquor still from Prohibition days and a more defined Confederate defense locale. Travel a boardwalk over a freshwater marsh and consider what life was like back when the Old Ferry Road led to a landing where locals would boat to Savannah to trade. Now this area, once home to the giant ground sloth, is a pocket of nature on an island of growth in a sea of civilization.

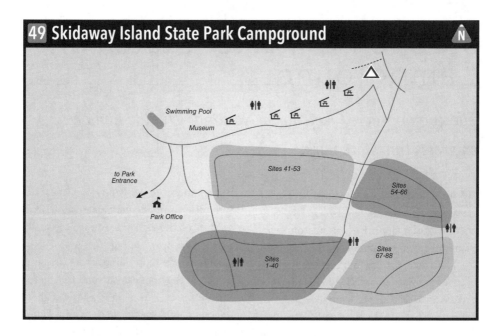

49 Skidaway Island State Park Campground

- Sites 41-53
- Sites 54-66
- Sites 1-40
- Sites 67-88
- Swimming Pool
- Museum
- to Park Entrance
- Park Office

:: Getting There

From Exit 94 on I-95, take GA 204 East 10.5 miles, then turn right on the GA 204 Spur. Stay on the GA 204 Spur 7 miles and turn left into the signed park road to enter the park after 0.25 miles.

GPS COORDINATES   N31° 57' 4.42"   W81° 03' 6.46"

50

Stephen C. Foster State Park Campground

The 400,000-acre Okefenokee National Wildlife Refuge encircles this state park.

The **Okefenokee Swamp** is one of Georgia's natural jewels. Luckily, Stephen C. Foster State Park stands on Jones Island, nearly in the middle of the Okefenokee. From here, you can tour the swamp along 25 miles of waterways with your own boat or a rental or go on a ranger-led cruise. Much of the swamp outside the state park lies within the boundaries of the Okefenokee Swamp National Wildlife Refuge. Here, the emphasis is on wildlife, chief among them alligators. Besides gators, the refuge includes more than 50 species of reptiles, 200 bird species, and nearly 50 types of mammals, spread over cypress-lined waterways, an occasional pine- and oak-covered island, and in open marshes where water lilies bloom.

Don't be discouraged by the presence of cable hookups in the campground. This normally spells RVs and would merit exclusion from this book, but not here. The campground is divided into two loops. Area I is along a winding, paved road with many good tent sites situated beneath a forest of

:: Ratings

BEAUTY: ★ ★ ★
PRIVACY: ★ ★ ★
SPACIOUSNESS: ★ ★
QUIET: ★ ★ ★ ★
SECURITY: ★ ★ ★ ★ ★
CLEANLINESS: ★ ★ ★

tall pines and live oaks. Palmetto bushes and wax myrtle form adequate campsite barriers. Most of the sites are average to small, which keeps away the big rigs. Area II is a longer, narrower loop. Some of the sites here are open to the noonday sun and have grass campsite floors. This area is a little higher, more piney, and drier in times of rain. Thick brush separates most sites. The end of the loop offers pull-through sites for the big rigs.

March is a good time to visit, before the spring crowds and the mosquitoes arrive. The campground fills the entire month of April. Fall can be excellent, though the skeeters may still be a bit troublesome. Call ahead for a bug report. Winter is quiet, and mild days can be a treat. Summer is too hot and buggy. A small camp store has limited supplies. Bring everything you can, as the nearest full-service grocery store is 45 miles away. Also, check ahead about park gate closure times. The wildlife refuge is strictly gated; if the gate is closed, it stays closed until morning.

The drainage pattern is an interesting aspect of this wide and shallow catch basin that is the Okefenokee. Though located near the Atlantic Ocean, most of the water flows out the Suwannee River, which can be followed downstream directly from the park all the way to the Gulf of Mexico. Another, smaller portion of the flow exits to the Atlantic via the St. Mary's River. For the park visitor,

:: Key Information

ADDRESS: Route 1, Box 131, Fargo, GA 31631

OPERATED BY: Georgia State Parks

CONTACT: 912-637-5274, **gastateparks .org;** reservations 800-864-7275, **reserveamerica.com**

OPEN: Year-round

SITES: 68

SITE AMENITIES: Picnic table, fire ring, water, electricity, cable TV hookup

ASSIGNMENT: First come, first served or by reservation

REGISTRATION: At park office

FACILITIES: Hot showers, flush toilets

PARKING: At campsites only

FEE: $25 tent, $30 others

ELEVATION: 120 feet

RESTRICTIONS

■ **Pets:** On leash only
■ **Fires:** In fire rings only
■ **Alcohol:** At campsites only
■ **Vehicles:** None
■ **Other:** 14 day stay-limit

these waterways offer paddling and boating opportunities galore. Be apprised that the waterways lie within the national wildlife refuge, which requires an additional entrance fee beyond that of the state park. Here, you can follow the 3-mile Day-Use Canoe Trail, or head to Billy's Island, where a boat dock makes landing your craft easy. Once on the island, you can take the Billy's Island Walking Trail, which makes a loop from the dock.

Many folks, especially those with motorboats, like to tool up to Minnie's Lake and Big Water Lake. Big Water Lake is a popular fishing destination. Chain pickerel—or jackfish as they are known locally—are the prime game fish. On my first trip into the swamp, my paddling partner, Wes Shepherd, caught a jackfish almost immediately. As he was reeling it in, an alligator came over to bite the fish off the line. Wes hurriedly reeled his line, then boldly grabbed the jackfish by the lip to pull it out of the water before the alligator could reach it. When he grabbed, he got a handful of sharp teeth! Handle jackfish with care while unhooking them from the line. Others will be fishing for more user-friendly bream, mudfish, and catfish. A fish-cleaning station

is conveniently located near the boat ramp for those inclined to eat their catch.

Boat tours run three times a day and are the easiest, most informative initiation to the swamp. You can also rent johnboats with a motor, or a canoe for a quieter experience. Many campers who bring their own boats opt for kayaks, an efficient way to see more of the area. Other visitors use the park as a jumping-off point for extended overnight trips into the refuge. Permits are required for backcountry trips.

If you want to stay on land, take the Pine Uplands Trail. It explores the towering evergreen forests that occupy much of what is not water in these parts. And land is at a premium here. The park nature trail travels on land and over a 2,100-foot boardwalk into the swamp. Before doing any of this, consider checking out the park interpretive center and museum. Here, you can learn about the natural and cultural history of the park. See the tools that both settlers and aboriginal inhabitants used. Other information ties together the web of life that is being preserved here in the Okefenokee. Park naturalists host interpretive programs on weekends, furthering your knowledge of the Peach State.

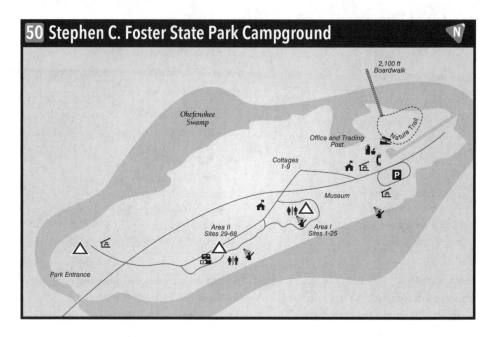

:: Getting There

From Fargo, just south of the Suwannee River, take GA 177 North 17 miles to end at the state park.

GPS COORDINATES N30° 49' 15.25" W82° 22' 1.59"

APPENDIX A

• • • • • • • • • • • • • • • • • • • •

Camping Equipment Checklist

Except for the large and bulky items on this list, I keep a plastic storage container full of the essentials for car camping so they're ready to go when I am. I make a last-minute check of the inventory, resupply anything that's low or missing, and away I go.

COOKING UTENSILS

Bottles of salt, pepper, spices, sugar, cooking oil, and maple syrup in waterproof, spill-proof containers
Can and bottle openers
Corkscrew
Cups, plastic or tin
Dish soap (biodegradable), sponge, towel
Flatware
Food of your choice
Frying pan, spatula
Fuel for stove
Lighter, matches in waterproof container
Plates
Pocketknife
Fire starter
Pot with lid
Stove
Tin foil
Wooden spoon

FIRST-AID KIT

Antibiotic cream
Aspirin or ibuprofen
Band-Aids
Diphenhydramine (Benadryl)
Gauze pads
Insect repellent
Moleskin
Sunscreen/lip balm
Tape, waterproof adhesive
Tweezers

SLEEPING GEAR

Pillow
Sleeping bag
Sleeping pad, inflatable or insulated
Tent with ground tarp and rainfly

MISCELLANEOUS

Bath soap (biodegradable), washcloth, and towel
Camp chair
Candles
Cooler
Deck of cards
Flashlight/headlamp
GPS
Lantern
Maps (road, trail, topographic, etc.)
Paper towels
Plastic zip-top bags
Smart phone
Sunglasses
Toilet paper
Water bottle
Wool blanket

OPTIONAL

Barbecue grill
Binoculars
Field guides on bird, plant, and wildlife identification
Fishing rod and tackle box

APPENDIX B

● ●

Sources of Information

CHATTAHOOCHEE-OCONEE NATIONAL FORESTS
1755 Cleveland Hwy.
Gainesville, GA 30501
770-297-3000
www.fs.usda.gov/conf

GEORGIA DEPARTMENT OF TOURISM
P.O. Box 1776
Atlanta, GA 30301-1776
800-VISIT GA (847-4842)
exploregeorgia.org

GEORGIA STATE PARKS
2600 Hwy. 155 SW, Suite C
Stockbridge, GA 30281
404-656-2770, reservations 800-864-7275
gastateparks.org

U.S. ARMY CORPS OF ENGINEERS, MOBILE DISTRICT
P.O. Box 2288
Mobile, AL 36628-0001
251-471-5966
www.sam.usace.army.mil

INDEX

● ●

S

T

U

V

W